Living
FOOD ALLERGIES

Alex Gazzola

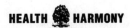
HEALTH HARMONY

An imprint of

B. Jain Publishers (P) Ltd.

An ISO 9001 : 2000 Certified Company

USA — EUROPE — INDIA

LIVING WITH FOOD ALLERGIES

First Edition: 2010
1st Impression: 2010

© 2009 by Alex Gazzola

For sale within Asia & Africa only

Published by Kuldeep Jain for

HEALTH 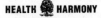 HARMONY

An imprint of
B. JAIN PUBLISHERS (P) LTD.
An ISO 9001 : 2000 Certified Company
1921/10, Chuna Mandi, Paharganj, New Delhi 110 055 (INDIA)
Tel.: +91-11-4567 1000 • *Fax:* +91-11-4567 1010
Email: info@bjain.com • *Website:* **www.bjainbooks.com**

Printed in India by
J.J. Offset Printers

ISBN: 978-81-319-0846-4

Acknowledgements

Those working in the field of allergy, be it in healthcare, research or support are, as I learned while researching this book, extremely overstretched. Therefore I'm especially grateful to those who responded to my enquiries and gave generously of what I suspect they had least to give, their time.

Thanks, then, to Aleks Kinay of the Latex Allergy Support Group; Professor John Warner of the University of Southampton; Carol Rae, Lindsey McManus, Muriel Simmons and all at Allergy UK; allergy dietitian Tanya Wright of Amersham Hospital, Buckinghamshire; Dr Clare Mills of the Institute of Food Research, Norwich, UK; Dr Mahesh PA, Associate Professor, JSSMC, and Director, Allergy Asthma Associates, Mysore, India; and Dr Taraneh Dean of the David Hide Asthma and Allergy Research Centre, Isle of Wight, UK.

Particular gratitude to Moira Austin, David Reading and all at the Anaphylaxis Campaign, UK.

Thanks due also to Phillip Hodson, Paul McGee, and Dr Rebecca Knibb of the University of Derby, UK, each of whose ideas and expertise formed much of Chapter 6; Fiona Marshall; pharmacist Maeve O'Connell; Joanne Williams for her observations on OAS; and all food allergy sufferers or those working in food allergy who have knowingly or otherwise contributed to this book.

Author's note: A previous, edited version of this book, Living with Food Allergy, was originally published by Sheldon Press in the UK.

Disclaimer: This book is designed to be a helpful and supportive resource for those who suffer from or care for people with food allergies, but cannot be used to diagnose or treat any medical disease, or act as a substitute for professional medical advice. Consult your doctor if you have or suspect you have a medical condition.

Introduction

The Food Allergy Problem

We are guilty of having become a little careless with the word 'allergy' in the 21st century. Many of us now casually describe ourselves as being 'a bit allergic' to some modern irritant such as household paint, fragrances or tobacco while someone of an idle disposition should perhaps not be surprised to hear himself jokingly diagnosed with a 'work allergy'.

But when pressed, most people are unsure of what allergy actually is. The sometimes careless media coverage of the subject may be in part responsible, as it might be for the increased number of people self diagnosing their 'allergies'. Inaccurate diagnosis by alternative therapists, many of whom misuse the word 'allergy', have added to the problem. We may not fully understand what it means to be allergic, yet many of us seem to think we are.

Allergies are serious conditions involving unwanted responses of the immune system. Whether sufferers react to pollen, insect stings or rubber latex, for instance, the symptoms such as nasal irritation (rhinitis), nettle rash (urticaria), eczema can be worrying. At worst, as with asthma, anaphylaxis and anaphylactic shock (allergic collapse) they have the potential to take someone's life.

Worldwide there is a severe allergy problem. In many Western nations, rates of allergy are at around 40% of the population, or sometimes even higher. Surprisingly, India is not far behind, with around 25% of the population now having at least one allergic condition. Most developing nations, increasingly adopting a Western lifestyle, are noticing increased rate of allergic diseases across varied age groups, especially the young.

In the medical world, sadly, allergy receives very little attention, with a lack of any national allergy programme in most developing nations, and fragmented medical care of variable quality. A lot of allergy medication is unavailable in parts of Asia and Africa, especially in rural areas. Much of the information we have about allergy is drawn from Western studies and research, but this is not always suitable to Indian, Asian or African healthcare. Although there are many similarities, allergies experienced in the tropical and developing nations can be very different.

This book is concerned with food allergy – an inappropriate, usually rapid and occasionally potentially life threatening response of the body's immune system towards a food component which is harmless to most other people.

Food allergy can cause great misery and worry. But because many mistakenly describe themselves as food allergic, the seriousness of the condition can be underestimated, with friends and family members, catering workers, even doctors, all sometimes sceptical about genuine cases. If you're really allergic to food, the world can seem unsympathetic.

Estimates of sufferers worldwide vary, but the West is badly affected. In Europe, up to 8% of children and 4% of adults have a food allergy, with figures perhaps still rising, while in the US, peanut allergy alone affects around 7% of individuals. To some extent because of the issues described above, we do not have accurate figures about the number of people affected in developing nations. However, it is thought that upto 3% of Indians may have food allergies, the majority under 40 years of age. Food allergies cause roughly 30,000 emergency treatments and 100 to 200 deaths per year in the nation. Up to 3 million Indians may have peanut allergy alone. The situation in African and other Asian nations is worsening too.

If the increased tendency to adopt Western lifestyle continues, and we don't address the problem with research and education, there is no reason to suppose this is a problem which is going to go away, and no reason to imagine that the rise in sufferers will not continue.

How this book will help

'*Living with Food Allergies*' aims to inform, support and empower sufferers and their families to cope with everything from the day-to-day practicalities of dealing with the condition to the long term implications of allergic illness triggered by food.

Food safety, diet and nutrition are obvious concerns, and these are considered thoroughly. The psychological impact of food allergy is given very little consideration, so chapter 7 is here to address the imbalance. Oral Allergy Syndrome, an increasingly common condition, usually directly related to hay fever, is another topic about which there is little information, and this is covered in depth too. The comprehensive Useful Resources section will be valuable to those seeking practical solution to problems.

Although they are not food allergies, the subject of food intolerances is covered briefly in Appendix 1. These include lactose intolerance (inability to digest the sugar in milk), coeliac disease (a digestive disorder, triggered by wheat and related grains) and other non allergic reactions to foods or food ingredients. A more detailed examination of the subject is provided by the book 'Living with Food Intolerance' (Sheldon Press), by the same author.

This book mostly assumes that the reader is the adult food allergy sufferer. However, most of the general information also applies to children and teenagers. Issues of interest to parents such as advice on attending school are covered too, and when the recommendations and information concerning various age groups differ, this is clearly pointed out in the text.

The book is not specifically intended for parents of allergic babies or very young children, although there is plenty of helpful information for these groups too including about prevention of allergy. Bear in mind, though, that the diagnosis, management, treatment and prognosis of food allergy in the very young can be specific to that age group, so while some information will be valid, some advice may be unsuited to babies.

This book is probably best read if the reader or the reader's child has already been diagnosed through orthodox means usually via a doctor and allergy consultant rather than through a high street test or alternative therapist. Testing for food allergy is covered in Appendix 2. However, it is hoped it may be of use to anyone who suspects they or one of their children may have a food allergy, families and friends of those with allergies, health and nutrition professionals, teachers and anyone with an interest in this important subject.

Publisher's Note

Knowing the term 'allergy' vaguely is not enough, we must know more about the matter. The author warns the masses that by adopting more and more artificial lifestyle and western style of development, we are in a way increasing the cases of allergy. People don't take their allergies seriously and tend to self diagnose their problem. Moreover, inaccurate diagnosis by alternative therapists adds to the problem. Symptoms could range from nasal irritation, nettle rash to anaphylactic shock in worse cases. The main aim to publish this book is to inform, support and empower sufferers and their families to cope with this condition which if not seriously taken could prove to be life threatening.

Information given in this book covers detailed description regarding causes, symptoms, diagnosis, treatment and management. I wish this comes out to be a useful tool for all those people suffering with food allergies, as well as health and nutrition professionals.

Kuldeep Jain
C.E.O., B. Jain Publishers (P) Ltd.

About the Author

Alex Gazzola is an author, journalist, researcher and writing tutor who has written widely on health, food and nutritional issues over a career span of twelve years. He has a special interest in food sensitivities, allergies and digestion, and his previous book, *Living with Food Intolerance*, is published by Sheldon Press in the UK (www.sheldonpress.com). His work has appeared in The Guardian and The Times (UK), The Sunday Telegraph (Australia), Business Day (South Africa) and the Hindu (India), and around 120 other publications in 20 countries. His website is www.alexgazzola. co.uk

Contents

Chapter 1

What is Food Allergy?

A food allergic reaction is a prompt, inappropriate and adverse response towards an otherwise harmless food component which is triggered by your immune system, the body of cells responsible for defending you from infection.

The substance responsible for a food allergy is called a food allergen. Typically, this allergen is a type of protein, for instance, one of the many proteins found in nuts or fish which your immune system mistakenly believes to be a threat. The allergen enters your body through the delicate membranes of the mouth, through the skin, or when you swallow it. If you're particularly sensitive, inhaling airborne particles of the culprit food can trigger a reaction, the allergen gaining access through your respiratory system.

Symptoms which vary according to several factors include tingling in the mouth, a runny nose, rashes, wheezing and asthma, swelling of the mouth and throat, and vomiting.

Allergic sensitization

For your immune system to 'decide' that a protein is dangerous to your body, it must previously have been exposed to it and subsequently have developed sensitization to it.

Sensitization is an over reaction of your immune system to what it perceives as an 'invader'. Anxious to protect the body, the immune system can respond to a new and suspect protein by manufacturing molecules called antibodies to tackle it.

The antibodies usually involved in food allergies are called Immunoglobulin E (IgE). Once they are formed, IgE antibodies attach themselves to immune cells called mast cells, which tend to be found where your body is most vulnerable to invasion from microbes such as the nose and lung.

When you then come into contact with allergens to which you've been sensitized, the allergen and its corresponding IgE antibody bind together. This binding causes the mast cell to be activated and release inflammatory chemicals such as histamine.

Problems occur when the volume of released inflammatory chemicals causes unwanted changes in the body. These include the typical symptoms of food allergies like swelling, rashes, diarrhoea and vomiting all aimed at flushing out the 'invader'. Unfortunately for you, these reactions can be uncomfortable, distressing and at worst life threatening.

Age and sensitization

Allergic sensitization often happens when very young, before the immune system is mature enough to deal with the complex proteins typically associated with food allergies. A child can be fed an allergen directly, consume it in the mother's breast milk. There is even some evidence that creams used in infancy containing food proteins such as nappy creams can occasionally sensitize children to the source food, though this is probably very rare.

Increasingly, however, sensitization or the emergence of food allergy symptoms in young adulthood and in later life is becoming more common, for reasons which are unclear. Sometimes, in food industry workers, occupational exposure is to blame, for instance, those working in flour factories and exposed to inhaled allergens may become sensitized and later react to wheat.

The allergic march

This refers to the progress of allergic disease through life in susceptible young children. It typically begins with eczema in the early months of life and this may indicate a food allergy. Food allergies tend to appear in the early years of a child's life and as children get older, asthma and allergies to pets and dust mites may also develop, as well as pollen allergy (hay fever) a little later.

However, following sensitization, the progression of allergic illness through life is difficult to predict.

Childhood food allergies can disappear permanently, diminish in severity, remain unchanged, or diminish or disappear then re-emerge in adulthood, sometimes in a new form. Most young children outgrow sensitivities to milk, eggs, wheat and soy by the age of five, for instance, but only about one in five will outgrow sensitivities to nuts. Fish allergy also tends to be kept into adulthood, although it is fairly uncommon in childhood.

Food allergies which start later in life are more likely to be permanent problems which tend not to worsen, and in some cases may improve.

However, it is important to stress that food allergies and food allergic reactions are extremely unpredictable by their nature.

Causes

Although we understand how people become sensitised and allergic to food, the reasons for this remain unclear.

What we do know is that some are more susceptible than others to food allergies, and this is due to atopy – the hereditary and genetic predisposition to suffer from any allergic illness. Typical allergic diseases include pollen allergy (hay fever), eczema and asthma.

If you suffer from allergies other than food allergies, or if your parents suffered from any allergic conditions, it is more likely that you will develop food allergies, and more likely that your children will too. That said, most individuals with allergic tendencies do not develop food allergies, and some non-atopic people and those from non-atopic families do (especially in infancy).

Other factors

There are undoubtedly considerations other than genetic to take into account, given that studies on identical twins show they often show different allergic status. Several ideas have been suggested, and a combination may be at work.

The hygiene hypothesis

This is the idea that because of our modern aversion to dirt and our tendency to disinfect our homes too much, we are no longer exposing ourselves to the largely safe everyday bacteria which are thought to safely exercise the immune system's protective mechanisms. In the absence of such helpful triggers, the immune system instead turns its attention towards other 'intruders' such as food proteins. Those brought up in natural, rural environments, exposed daily to outdoor and natural life, show lower incidences of allergy than people brought up in clean city homes.

Smaller families

With couples now tending to have smaller families, children are less likely to be exposed to infections 'brought home' by older siblings as would have occurred in previous generations with larger families. Reduced sharing of childhood infections could again be resulting in under exercised immune systems which are more likely to malfunction.

Altered gut bacteria

According to research, allergic children have lower levels of beneficial or 'probiotic' bacteria in their intestines. It's uncertain whether this may be a likely cause or consequence of allergy, but it has been suggested that the use of too many antibiotics has unbalanced our internal ecosystems, possibly affecting immunity.

Altered nutrition

Some researchers feel that our modern tendency to eat less fruit and vegetables and more Western processed foods and meals could be leaving us lacking in some nutrients. This could also be exposing us to more proteins (and therefore more potential food triggers).

Furthermore, foods previously unknown to us are now nothing more than an air flight away, with an array of exotic and foreign foods being imported and available at many supermarkets and shops, each with their own collection of allergens which we are not able to cope with.

Traces in our foods of pesticides, fertilisers and growth hormones used in modern farming practice may also be confusing the picture.

Pollutants, chemicals and smoking

Environmental pollution, household chemicals and toiletries, and exposure to tobacco smoke could all be harming normal immunological responses in some people.

Pollution could also be problematic for plants. The increase in allergy to fruits and vegetables may be due to plants producing greater amounts of allergenic proteins as a defence against greater environmental stresses.

The major allergens

Around 90% of food allergy reactions in Western children are caused by milk, eggs, wheat, soy, peanuts and tree nuts.

In adults, all types of nuts and seafood appear to be the biggest problem foods.

According to several sources, the most common food allergens often called 'the big eight' are the following:

1. Peanuts
2. Tree nuts (such as cashews and walnuts)
3. Fish
4. Shellfish, such as shrimp and lobster
5. Milk and dairy foods
6. Eggs (both yolk and white)
7. Wheat
8. Soya

While some of these foods (especially fish and shellfish) can be a problem in Asian and African countries, there are others which also frequently cause problems:

1. Legumes/daals, such as chickpeas/chana daal, peas, lentils, urad bean/black gram.
2. Seeds, spices and flavourings, such as sesame, poppy, sunflower, garlic and mustard.
3. Rice (which is very rare in the West).

Increasingly, throughout the world, raw (and occasionally cooked) fruits and vegetables are causing problems. Some of the most serious include bananas, apples and kiwi. Interestingly, each country or geographical area can have very specific, curious food allergies, sometimes related to their local climate or cuisine, for example,

1. Coconut (India)
2. Royal jelly (Hong Kong)
3. Bird's nest (Singapore)
4. Buckwheat (Japan)
5. Celery (Switzerland)
6. Pineapple (Ghana)
7. Corn/maize (Mexico and US)
8. Chestnuts (Korea)

Another key point to make is that it is perfectly possible to be mildly allergic to peanut, for instance, and dangerously allergic to a usually safe food, such as pear. There are around 200 foods on record which are known to have caused reactions, and of varying degrees of severity.

It is the same when it comes to the issue of cooked versus uncooked food. Roasting nuts, for instance, appears to increase their potential to cause allergies, and in the case of pecan nuts can even create new allergens.

Meanwhile, some people allergic to egg can tolerate processed eggs, and possibly hard boiled eggs, but not lightly cooked eggs. Some react to raw fish, some to cooked, and some to both.

Cooking or otherwise processing fruits and vegetables tend to make them less reactive although many who react to celery do so to both cooked and raw forms.

Non allergens

Although allergic reactions to most foods are possible, certain food components, many essential to our diet, do not cause them.

You cannot be allergic to the vitamin C or salt in a food, for instance, or any other vitamin or essential mineral. Neither can you be allergic to water, to fats or oils, to alcohol, or to simple sugars, such as table sugar, glucose or lactose (milk sugar).

It is proteins which cause the vast majority of food allergies. Reactions to non protein components are likely to be food intolerances or other unusual sensitivities (see Appendix 1).

Chapter 2

Symptoms and Reactions

Food allergic symptoms and reactions are many and varied, and can be localised (affecting one specific part or area of the body) or systemic (affecting many parts or areas of the body).

Localised reactions are confined to the point of contact with the allergen; with food, this is usually the lips, mouth and throat.

Systemic or whole body reactions are usually more dangerous.

Food allergy symptoms tend to be acute, that is, they come on rapidly, are sharp and relatively short lived. Chronic allergic illness which is of gradual onset, slow progression, and long lasting is only rarely triggered by allergies to food, but more commonly can be worsened by them.

Reactions of the skin

Urticaria is the most common acute food allergic reaction of the skin. It is a rash characterised by raised swellings called wheals, itchiness, and reddening or flushing, occurring within minutes of exposure to the culprit food. Also called hives or nettle rash, urticaria is brought on by histamine release into the skin's layers, causing fluid to seep from microscopic blood vessels into the skin's tissues. Food allergy is unlikely to be involved in chronic urticaria. Urticaria can also be triggered by extremes of temperature, sun exposure, pressure, toiletries and cosmetics.

Around half of acute urticarial food reactions are accompanied by angioedema or localised swelling or puffiness which occurs when blood vessel leakage is more severe. Acute angioedema in the absence of urticaria is possible, but uncommon. Chronic angioedema, a serious symptom, is unlikely to be food allergic in origin.

Eczema or atopic dermatitis is a chronic inflammatory and itchy, and sometimes flaky, weepy and scaly skin conditions, particularly prevalent in the young, and often associated with other allergic disorders such as asthma. Food allergy, quite often egg allergy, can make eczema worse, but is very unlikely to be the underlying cause. Other factors such as toiletries, pets and dust mites and environmental conditions are also common irritants in eczema.

Reactions of the respiratory system

Inflammation of the mucous membranes of the nose, called rhinitis, is a common, minor food allergic response, while a runny nose, called rhinorrhoea, is a symptom of increased nasal secretion. Both are more likely when culprit foods are inhaled or sniffed rather than consumed. Bloodshot, watery eyes (allergic conjunctivitis) and sneezing may also occur. Chronic rhinitis or perennial allergic rhinitis is associated with pollens, dust mites, moulds or pets.

Wheezing and shortness of breath are symptoms of asthma, a narrowing of the bronchial airways in the lung caused by inflammation, which can occur in more serious food allergic responses, especially in chronic asthma or otherwise atopic patients. Wheezing may be caused or exacerbated by angioedema in the throat. Chronic asthma may be caused or worsened by food allergy, but other factors such as environmental pollution, tobacco, exercise and pets are more likely.

Reactions of the gastrointestinal system

Nausea, abdominal pain and vomiting can be symptoms of food allergy when the food culprits cause internal irritation and inflammation of the gullet/foodpipe (oesophagus) and stomach. Although there are other causes of such symptoms like bacteria, poisons, and vomiting in combination with skin or respiratory symptoms implies a severe allergic reaction.

Anaphylaxis

Of all the allergic reactions, anaphylaxis is the most extreme.

Food allergic reactions considered above can be and normally are all involved, but anaphylactic reactions progress further. Typical symptoms of food induced anaphylaxis, approximately in the order they usually present themselves, include some but certainly not necessarily all of the following:

1. Flushing, itching and urticaria, especially around the face and mouth initially, then often progressing elsewhere on the body.
2. Swelling (oedema), especially around the face, oral area and throat but potentially more widespread.
3. A blocked nose and sneezing.
4. Hoarseness and difficulty speaking.
5. Wheeziness and laboured breathing (more pronounced in asthmatics).
6. Difficulty swallowing.
7. An increased pulse or palpitations (tachycardia).
8. Gastric pain, nausea, vomiting.

9. A sense of impending doom; anxiety, panic, confusion, disorientation.
10. Lower abdominal pain, diarrhoea, incontinence.
11. Weakness, dizziness and 'floppiness', caused by a sudden drop in blood pressure.
12. Circulatory collapse and unconsciousness, the anaphylactic shock.

Anaphylactic reactions usually come on rapidly, within minutes or even seconds of exposure or rarely quite slowly, up to an hour or more later. Also, the progression from mild oral symptoms to dangerous respiratory and cardiovascular breakdown can be extremely quick, or less typically much slower. There can be a lot of variation.

Older children and adults are more likely to suffer from anaphylaxis, it is less likely to affect babies and very young children. Even a trace quantity of almost any food can cause it; the main culprits are listed on pg. 6, but peanuts and tree nuts, and fish and shellfish, are undoubtedly the prime danger foods.

Risk factors

Anaphylaxis can kill through asphyxiation because of swelling of the throat, cardiac arrest and circulatory collapse, or a fatal asthma attack. So how do you know whether you're at risk?

Some doctors consider anyone allergic to tree nuts, peanuts, seeds and seafood no matter how mild their symptoms, to be at potential risk.

If you've had severe allergic responses in the past, this can also increase your chances of suffering an anaphylactic reaction. The same applies if you're asthmatic, in which case your food allergic reaction is more likely to be life threatening.

Having exercised before exposure can also turn a moderate

reaction into an anaphylactic one. Sometimes, exercise following a particular food even as long as a day later can be directly responsible for triggering a reaction. This rare condition is called exercise induced anaphylaxis and the cause can be difficult to pinpoint because no reaction is experienced from exposure to the allergen in the absence of exercise. Prawns/shrimp, celery and wheat (gluten) are some of the foods implicated in exercise induced anaphylaxis; the condition appears to be commonest in young female athletes.

Exposure to extremes of heat or cold can worsen a reaction. In some people, having taken aspirins or other drugs can exacerbate the reaction too. A high dose of the culprit allergen, perhaps when 'disguised' in an unfamiliar food can push a reaction over the edge, and if alcohol is involved, the reaction will be speedier, and your response time and judgement may be impaired.

Unfortunately, there have been a number of cases where anaphylactic reactions have occurred with absolutely no previous warning whatsoever. Sadly, susceptibility to anaphylaxis is normally lifelong. Other allergens which can cause anaphylaxis include insect stings, snake bites, latex (rubber), and drugs such as penicillin.

Anaphylactic reactions, like all other types of allergic reactions respond to prompt and appropriate treatment, which we look at in the next chapter.

Cross Reactions

When you are sensitised to a particular allergen and you react to it, it is also possible to react to other unrelated allergens which share similar characteristics. These responses, where previous sensitisation to one allergen results in symptoms emerging in response to others are known as cross reactions. The sensitzer does not necessary have to be a food allergen.

Oral Allergy Syndrome (OAS)

This is a particular type of food allergy to fruits, vegetables, herbs, spices, seeds and nuts which is restricted to the oral area, that is, the lips, the mouth, the tongue and sometimes the throat. It is very common in western nations but is fairly rare in developing nations at present, although this may change in future.

OAS only occurs in people with seasonal allergic rhinitis, more commonly known as hay fever. This is an allergy to one or more spores or pollens, such as grass pollens. The symptoms of hay fever include sneezing, running eyes and nose, itchy nose and occasionally light wheezing, headache and tiredness.

The proteins in pollens which cause reactions in hay fever are also present in many plant foods. When people with OAS eat some of these plant foods, their immune systems are confused into 'thinking' they are actually eating pollen, and so they experience reactions. Because of this, OAS is also called pollen food syndrome. It is not known how many people with hay fever may be affected in this way.

Itching and tingling in the mouth are the major symptoms of OAS if a trigger food is eaten, usually within minutes of consumption. There may be urticaria and angioedema around the mouth and throat if a larger portion of food is consumed. Usually it is only raw foods which pose a problem. In many cases, cooked or processed food do not trigger a reaction, because the allergens involved are very fragile and easily broken down by heat and processing.

However, merely preparing raw food can trigger mild breathing or eye symptoms if you're exposed to traces of vaporised juices, and peeling fruit and vegetables can bring on urticaria on the hands too. Wheezing is possible if the irritation and swelling spreads to the throat. However, the symptoms are not normally life threatening. Infact, they can be so mild that sufferers may ignore or barely be conscious of them.

Since the allergenic food proteins usually break down on contact with the stomach's digestive juices, reactions such as vomiting or stomach pain are very unlikely in OAS.

Incidence and prevalence

Hay fever is seasonal and you will only experience its symptoms when relevant plants or trees are pollinating in your part of the world. In India, the two principal pollen seasons run from February to April (tree pollens), and September to December (grass pollens and weed pollens such as parthenium). While, in Africa, the seasons run approximately from August through to April (grass pollens) and August to November (tree and weed pollens).

However, once you are sensitised to pollens, any associated food allergic cross reactions will occur all year round although out of the pollen season they are usually milder, and during the pollen season they are stronger.

Pollen related OAS is rare in children, but more frequently seen in older teenagers and young adults. Often, there is improvement in middle age and beyond.

In India, around one in seven of the population has allergic rhinitis, but it is unknown how many of these people suffer from related oral allergies.

Unfortunately, it is possible to become sensitized to a non native pollen during a foreign trip in peak hay fever season. For instance, someone with allergic tendencies from India visiting northern or central Europe during February to April can become sensitized to the birch tree pollen which is very common to that geographical area. Returning home, the person will not experience hay fever symptoms (there are no birch trees in India) but they may suffer food cross reactions to fruits such as jackfruit and apple.

Note that although pollen food reactions tend not to be serious, if you suffer from an allergy to a fruit, vegetable or nut in the absence of any pollen sensitivity, the reactions are more likely to be severe. For instance, apple allergies related to hay fever are less of a threat than apple allergies unrelated to hay fever.

It is rare that OAS progresses to anaphylaxis. Only 2% of sufferers have reported an episode, and these have typically involved nuts, celery, apple, strawberry or kiwi.

Types of Pollen Food Cross Reactions

Many vegetables and fruits can be involved.

Reactions are still being recorded and discovered, so this list cannot be complete, and can only give an idea of some of the foods that may be found to be a problem in some cases. Individuals with OAS often come across new foods to which they react, although some people only react to one or two and can safely eat all others without any problems or reactions. Any foods you do react to suggest that you're more likely to also react to close family members of the food. See Appendix 3 for further information on food families, but that does not necessarily mean you should be fearful of all foods in any category.

Tree pollens

People with allergies to tree pollens can potentially have oral allergies to many foods including avocado, members of the carrot family (carrots, coriander), the legume family (all daals, such as beans and lentils), the nightshade family (pepper, potato), pineapple, kiwi, the rose family (apple, pear; peach, plum), spinach, and many nuts and spices.

Grass pollens

It seems not many people sensitive to grass pollen have OAS, but reported reactions include to apple, kiwi, orange, peanut, daals and grass grains (such as wheat).

Weed pollens

Reactions to apple, the carrot family, the daisy family (camomile, sunflower seeds) and the melon family (melon, cucumber) are possible, as are those to spices (black pepper, poppy seed), and banana.

Other cross reactions

Apart from pollens, there are other sensitizers which can cross react with foods.

Mould spores

If you have allergic rhinitis which is not seasonal and occurs throughout the year (perennial), it could be caused by either internal or external mould or fungi spores. People who suffer from this allergy sometimes find that they react with mushrooms and edible fungi, as well as to yeast based spreads, or highly fermented or matured foods.

Bird feathers

A cross reaction in those allergic to bird feathers is possible with egg yolk.

Dust mites

The droppings of the house dust mite are very allergenic, and many people react to them. Asthma and eczema can be aggravated by them, and rhinitis is a common symptom. Occasionally, sufferers can react, sometimes severely, to kiwi, papaya/pawpaw, soy and especially shellfish such as shrimp, due to some unusual similarities between certain allergens present in both. (Although not a cross reaction, another danger is the consumption of dust mite contaminated flour, a common problem in Asian nations, which can lead to unpleasant reactions in those allergic to them. This is sometimes mistaken for allergy to the flour, rather than the mites.)

Cockroaches

This is a common indoor pest in Asian countries, and proteins found in cockroach saliva and feces are very allergenic. As with dust mites, people allergic to cockroaches can sometimes experience reactions when consuming shellfish and other seafood.

Latex

Allergy to latex (natural rubber) is common among healthcare workers regularly exposed to latex gloves, and others who work with latex. The condition is rare in the general population, but those undergoing a lot of surgery are at greater risk. Around half of those with latex allergy experience cross reactions with foods, which tend to be tropical fruits. Avocado appears to be the commonest culprit, followed by banana, chestnut and kiwi, but reactions to buckwheat, cherry, fig, mango, melon, papaya/pawpaw, passion fruit, peach, potato, tomato, nuts and daals are reported too and this list is growing. Reactions to latex and its cross reacting foods can be systemic and very serious.

Food-Food Cross Reactions

Of course foods regularly sensitize individuals, as is usually the case with the 'big eight', that is, peanuts, tree nuts, fish, shellfish, dairy, eggs, wheat and soy.

Allergies to one or more of these mean you're more likely to experience reactions to foods related to them. In the case of the legumes, soy and peanut, for instance, you may be more susceptible to other legumes such as gram (chana daal).

An allergy to wheat makes you more at risk of allergies to grains closely related to it, including barley and rye (a dark brown grain consumed mostly in eastern Europe).

Tree nuts and peanuts are unusual in that they are the best example of foods which tend to cross react with unrelated foods as well as to 'siblings'. Most tree nuts are not closely related, and yet becoming sensitized to one can make you vulnerable to reactions to others, and to peanut, which botanically speaking is a legume, not a nut. Equally, in reverse, sensitization to the peanut makes you not only more likely to react to other legumes, but to tree nuts too.

With most animal sourced foods, cross reactions are common. Sensitization to hen's eggs is likely to mean sensitization to all eggs as the culprit proteins are common to all types.

If you're allergic to cow's milk, there's a high likelihood you will react to other animal milks and there is also the possibility you will react to the same animal's meat. Infact, most children with beef allergy are also allergic to cow's milk, though it is less likely the other way around.

Similarly, if you've been sensitized to one fish, you're likely to experience reactions with at least several others; and it's a similar situation with crustaceans (crab, lobster, shrimp) and molluscs (clam, cockle, scallop).

Appendix 3 lists in detail plant and seafood families.

Chapter 3

Reaction Management

Obviously it is better to steer clear of your known triggers and in a few instances possibly other potentially troublesome foods, and chapters 4 and 5 will look closely at ways to avoid problem foods. Nevertheless, dealing with reactions is a fact of life, no matter how vigilant you or your child happen to be, so it is vital you learn how to best deal with them when they occur.

Although there is no cure for food allergy, there are medicines to help you manage reactions when they happen accidentally. Never take these before consuming a food to which you normally react or which cannot be guaranteed safe in the hope of preventing a reaction as this is potentially dangerous.

Antihistamines

Antihistamines counteract the effects of histamine, one of the principal chemicals released by the body during an allergic reaction.

Although antihistamines are known more for controlling allergic conditions such as hay fever, they can be effective in tackling the symptoms of mild food allergies. Many are available from a chemist and your doctor or pharmacist can advise on which may suit you or your child.

Loratadine (found in Loridin and Lormeg, for instance) and cetirizine (used in Zyrtec) are two which may be recommended. Both are non sedating, meaning they're unlikely to make you feel drowsy. Chlorpheniramine (used in Avil) is an older type of antihistamine, which can make some people drowsy. There are occasional advantages to sleep inducing antihistamines, for instance, if you suffer a mild reaction late in the evening which is likely to agitate you at a time when you're hoping to relax.

Most antihistamines come in tablet or liquid form. Tablets are easy to carry, but syrups can be taken without water. Syrups, usually sweetened, tend to be favoured by children, to whom a precise dose can be given. Some 'fast melt' antihistamines are now available, which simply dissolve in the mouth. In terms of performance, they are fairly similar.

Liquid antihistamines may be prescribed should you be at risk of anaphylaxis, but they are not enough to manage a systemic reaction, and in this case adrenaline is usually needed too (see p. 24).

Contraindications

Antihistamines may not suit everybody. For instance, if you have diabetes or a sugar intolerance, syrups may be inadvisable. Some antihistamines should not be taken by young children, so always seek advice when considering medication for your child. Those with decreased liver or kidney function and prostate enlargement must also seek advice. Pregnant or nursing women are often advised to avoid certain kinds; the safer ones tend to be the older varieties, but always speak to an expert for guidance.

Let your pharmacist know if you are taking other medicines

or have chronic or short term conditions. Groups who should be vigilant include epileptics, the elderly, glaucoma sufferers, asthmatics and those with cardiovascular disease or high blood pressure.

Some side effects are possible, including dry mouth, restlessness or headaches. Always read labels and leaflets carefully before taking antihistamines.

Asthma Inhalers

If you're asthmatic, you'll already have drugs to manage your condition. Asthma drugs are either preventers or relievers. Preventers counteract the inflammation in the lungs which triggers the contraction of the muscles surrounding the airways that causes asthmatic symptoms. Relievers relax those muscles, thereby opening up the airways, easing discomfort and breathing.

, Preventers should be taken as prescribed by your healthcare provider, but serve no direct purpose in treating acute food allergic reactions although the better your asthma is managed through preventative medication, the less severe any reactions are likely to be. If you feel your management of asthma is poor and could be improved upon, make an appointment with your doctor or consultant.

Relievers, though, in the form of inhalers (or bronchodilators) can help, and can be used in conjunction with antihistamines in the management of all allergic reactions to food.

Remember that symptoms of wheezing can signify a more serious reaction that may require adrenaline treatment, and that all adult and child asthmatics are more at risk.

Managing mild or OAS-related reactions

Experiencing mild symptoms, such as tingling and itching of the mouth, a minor rash, or itchy throat, which is characteristic of a mild food allergic reaction? Here's what to do:

1. Spit out any food at once, into your hand or preferably a cloth or napkin.
2. Rinse your mouth (and then eyes if necessary) thoroughly with plain water, taking someone with you if you use public facilities.
3. Drink some plain water if you can, to 'wash away' the food from your throat.
4. Take any medication such as antihistamines or inhalers, and keep them near to you.
5. If you're alone, stay close to a phone.
6. Rest, stay calm, and let the reaction pass, as it should within 30 minutes to an hour.
7. Do not panic or try to make yourself sick.
8. Keep your body cool, not warm, and relieve any mild heat rashes by fanning air onto affected areas and avoid scratching.
9. Use an eyewash if your eyes are irritated.
10. Avoid alcohol, taking exercise or hot baths in the hours after a reaction.
11. Later, review your management of the reaction – is there anything you could have done better?

Remember that OAS reactions are rarely dangerous, but if your reactions have been getting steadily worse, speak to your doctor or allergist.

Adrenaline

During an allergic reaction, the body's adrenal glands produce increased volumes of the hormone adrenaline (epinephrine). Adrenaline constricts your blood vessels, preventing them from leaking, and stopping your blood pressure from dropping too low;

it also stimulates your heart, relaxes the pulmonary muscles to improve your breathing, and helps reduce facial swelling.

However, during a rare, extreme reaction, the body can be so overwhelmed that its ability to produce enough adrenaline is compromised, which is why an adrenaline injection delivered into the thigh muscle can help stabilise life threatening symptoms until emergency services arrive to help.

Needle and Syringe

The simplest and cheapest way to provide adrenaline is through ampoules of adrenaline at the correct strength for you or for your child's age and size, which your doctor or allergist will advise you on and may prescribe to you. You will also be supplied with needles and syringes in order to draw out the suitable dose of adrenaline and administer it to yourself in the outer thigh. The general advice is to have a pre-prepared syringe of the correct dose with you at all times, and to change it every week to ensure the preparation you carry is sterile.

Although this is not the ideal equipment for administering adrenaline, this is often all that is available or affordable for patients in African and Asian nations.

Typical ampoules contain 0.5ml of 1:1000 adrenaline. The advice on doses varies considerably, so you must take your recommendations from your doctor, according to factors personal to you or your child.

A normal single adult dose is between 0.3ml and 0.5ml.

The recommended dose for children will vary depending on age and size. Children above 30kg or aged over 12 may well be advised to receive an adult dose.

For all children, the suggested dose is typically 0.01ml per kg of weight. For children weighing between 15kg and 30kg, therefore, the usual recommendation is a dose of between 0.15ml to 0.30ml.

A repeated dose is often recommended in all cases if there is no improvement or worsening of symptoms after five to ten minutes. About one in five anaphylactic episodes requires a second dose.

Auto-injector pens

Although these are not yet widely available throughout the developing world, this may hopefully change in future.

Auto-injector pens are one time use automated drug delivery systems, each containing a dose of the hormone adrenaline and a concealed, spring loaded needle. There are three major pens used in the West: the established EpiPen, the younger Anapen, and the very new Twinject.

All three come in adult and child doses. The dose in adult pens deliver a 0.3mg dose of adrenaline, the children's dose is 0.15mg which is suitable for children weighing between 30kg and 15kg (and sometimes less). Children weighing more than 30kg will usually be prescribed adult pens.

A difference between the three is in their method of use: the EpiPen requires a 'jabbing' motion to trigger its spring-loaded mechanism; the Anapen features a firing button; the Twinject requires users to press the pen into the thigh firmly.

Leaflets accompanying the pens give full details on their use, and video demonstrations on the relevant websites show how they can be safely employed when needed.

Deciding whether to use adrenaline

If you've experienced severe reactions previously, know you've been exposed to your trigger and symptoms have begun, most doctors would recommend that you use your adrenaline at once even while your symptoms may still be mild.

If you have no experience of an anaphylactic reaction but have been prescribed adrenaline as a precaution then distinguishing a mild food reaction and the onset of a serious reaction can be difficult. Often the initial symptoms are the same. Here are some questions to consider:

1. Do symptoms seem more severe than ever before and are they steadily worsening?
2. Are there signs of all over symptoms such as rashes or itchiness around the body?
3. Is your throat tightening and your voice hoarse, or are you coughing or choking?
4. Are you wheezing uncomfortably or experiencing asthma symptoms?
5. Are you experiencing difficulty breathing or swallowing?
6. Are you feeling sick, dizzy, weak or faint?
7. Do you have severe abdominal pain?

Each can signify the onset of an anaphylactic response, in which case you should use your adrenaline immediately.

If experience tells you, your symptoms seem to be mild and stable, take action appropriate to a mild reaction or as directed by your allergist or medical advisor, but stay alert to any worsening of your symptoms and ready to act accordingly.

If you are unsure, the general opinion is that you should use your adrenaline. The drug is safe, you are unlikely to feel pain from the needle, and you should not experience any long lasting side effects if you use it when not strictly necessary. The worse side effects seem to be short term like a 'rush of blood to the head' feeling, a heightened sense of stress or anxiety, sweating or shaking, and a stronger heartbeat. These will all pass.

If you think you may have been exposed to your allergen, but do not have symptoms yet, take some antihistamines and remain calm and alert. It is better not to inject unless and until symptoms begin, after all, it is possible you were not exposed to the allergen or even sufficient quantities of it, or much less likely that you have outgrown the allergy.

Using adrenaline

As soon as you realise you're having what appears to be the making of a serious allergic response, act immediately and never deny the problem, or question whether you're over reacting or making a fuss.

If you are with other people, tell them what is happening, take out your adernaline kit and ask someone to call medical emergency services and report that you are having a suspected allergic and anaphylactic reaction.

Use your adrenaline as directed or instructed. Then, massage the injected area for ten seconds. You should feel the benefits almost at once.

If you're feeling faint and light headed, it's usually better to lie on your back and raise your legs by propping them on a chair or against a wall, or get someone to hold them up in order to help get blood to your heart and head and raise your blood pressure. If you're feeling faint and sick, it's safer to lie on your side to eliminate the risk of choking on vomit.

If you have acute asthmatic symptoms, however, it's sometimes better to sit upright with your arms anchored so that your neck and shoulder muscles can be used for breathing. That said, it is far more important to sustain blood pressure than it is to deal with wheezing. Anaphylactic death from low blood pressure can be quick.

If you are alone, inject first and then call emergency services.

If you can, then call a friend or family member to join you. Note the time when they arrive, medical staff will need to know when you injected. Don't at any stage leap up off the floor if you've been lying down, only get up very slowly and carefully and lie back down if you still feel dizzy.

Remember, that adrenaline auto-injectors should be used only on the upper outer portion of the thigh, anywhere else on the body can be dangerous and that you can if necessary inject through most clothing, including denim.

An ordinary syringe and needle is best used on unclothed skin. Again it should be used in the thigh muscle.

After you use adrenaline

Remain calm. Take a dose of antihistamines if you can and haven't already and use your asthma reliever if you need to. There are no additional risks involved in using all three forms of medication in combination. Because the body rapidly eliminates adrenaline so you may need a second injection five to ten minutes after the first if symptoms don't improve, worsen suddenly or help is slow in arriving.

If it does not interfere with self treatment, which should be your priority, save a portion of the food which you feel triggered your response or better still, ask someone to put it aside or store it in a freezer if it's degradable, as you may need it later to identify the culprit.

When paramedics arrive, give used needles or pens to them. They will assess you, possibly give you more treatment and in all likelihood take you to Accident and Emergency.

At A&E, you'll be treated further, possibly with antihistamines, corticosteroids (which fight inflammation), adrenaline (via injection or a nebuliser) and in extreme cases oxygen and intravenous fluids.

Ideally, you'll be monitored for up to six hours. This is important, because repeat or 'rebound' or 'late phase' reactions called biphasic reactions can happen hours and even days after initial exposure. These occur when you have swallowed significant quantities of allergens which are resistant to breakdown in the body, such as peanut allergens, as they may continue to be absorbed through the digestive system for some time.

If you are discharged very early, ask to stay. If that's impossible due to bed or staff shortages, it's a good idea to remain on site in a waiting area for several hours. Be aware of the possibility of a secondary reaction and remember to obtain replacement adrenaline before you leave. You may also be given additional medication which you should take as directed.

After the reaction

Don't exert yourself. For several days avoid alcohol and temperature extremes (such as hot baths) and take as much rest as possible.

Once you're recovered, review what happened and your emergency response procedure. What didn't go smoothly? What can you improve? Is there anything you can learn in order to help you next time? Speak to your doctor or consultant or to other people with allergies or children with allergies for advice.

If the cause of the reaction remains a puzzle, it's important to find out how it occurred. This can be a time consuming task, but it's vital you pursue it until you get a definitive answer.

If you suspect a contaminant in a food product you thought was safe may have triggered your reaction, or that a manufacturer has made a packaging or labelling error, report it to the manufacturer and/or the store from which the product was bought. They will want to know packaging information, such as batch number, product code, place of purchase and expiry dates, so hold on to this.

If you suspect that you did not consume your particular allergen, you need to consider other possibilities including having developed a new allergy to another food. Appendix 3 on food families might suggest a possible cross reaction, or else speak to your doctor or allergist who may be able to deduce the culprit or suggest further tests to help identify it.

If you were dining at a restaurant, make an appointment to speak with the chef in order to carefully go through the ingredients of your meal, if only to eliminate the possibility of your having a previously unknown allergy.

Adrenaline care

Your adrenaline is a life saving medicine which you should treat with great care.

Firstly, and most essentially, always carry it with you. Most deaths due to anaphylaxis occur when adrenaline is not available for administration in the early stages of a reaction. Carry it in the same place always, so you and others, know where to find it. You can buy protective carrying cases for your adrenaline. See Useful resources.

Ask your doctor to write down instructions for using your adrenaline and if you have an auto-injector pen, read the instructions that come with it. Re-read these frequently to consolidate your understanding. Ask a nurse or doctor at your local medical centre to give you a refresher lesson from time to time.

Healthy adrenaline should be clear and colourless. If it's cloudy or yellow it should be replaced. If you have injector pens, check your adrenaline and its expiry date regularly. Adrenaline which is more than three months past its expiry will be ineffective. Users can register with manufacturers' date alert service to receive timely letter or e-mail reminders to have injectors replaced.

Adrenaline can degrade in hot or cold conditions, so protect it from direct sunlight or hot cars, and never store in the refrigerator or alongside ice. The idea is to keep it at comfortable room temperature but never too cold or too hot.

Friends and family

Everyone close to you needs to be made aware of your condition and the ways you manage it.

Don't overwhelm people at first. Think back to how it took you a while to get used to your diagnosis and medication and their implications, it's the same for your loved ones. 'Train' them gradually. For example, first make them aware of what your food allergy is, where your culprit may be hidden, and how even a trace amount can affect you if this is the case. Show them your medical jewellery, if you wear any.

You also need to tell them of the signs and symptoms of anaphylaxis, refer them to relevant sections of this book.

Then, show them your medication. When you think they're ready, introduce them to your emergency procedure and your adrenaline. It's important you do this, as knowing there are people looking out for you who can assist in an emergency is reassuring; most will be only too glad to help relieve some of the stress from you.

Auto-injector pen suppliers offer 'trainer' pens which are useful in demonstrating to friends and relatives how your pens work. These can also be useful to practise with. Trainer pens look very similar to the real thing, but do not have adrenaline or a needle. Manufactures have additional materials such as training packs with patient information and posters for your office and school. You can call or write to ask them.

Action plans

If you suffer such a serious reaction that you're unable to administer your own medication, others need to step in. If you are at risk of such a reaction, you must plan for this.

Apart from educating them through this book, other materials, and your own instruction it helps to give them an action plan of what to do in an emergency. Because each individual is different, an all suitable template is not appropriate. You should formulate a plan specific to you with the assistance of your doctor or allergy specialist.

An action plan could include:

1. Details of your allergy, your typical symptoms on exposure, and signs of an anaphylactic response.
2. How you should be positioned or assisted during a reaction.
3. How to check your airways, and how you can be helped with your breathing if you are struggling?
4. Where your medication, including your adrenaline, is kept, and how it should be used if you're unconscious?
5. An instruction to call the emergency services, and what they should be told. For instance, that a patient is suffering a suspected anaphylactic reaction, that adrenaline has been/ is being administered, the address of the patient's location (include on the sheet those of your home, study or workplace and anywhere else you commonly visit).
6. Follow up instructions, that someone should wait outside to direct emergency services, that a second injection can be administered after a specified time...

You should give this to everyone with whom you live or work closely and carry one yourself. Spend time going through it with people and be prepared to answer or find answers to questions. Feedback can be invaluable. If anything is unclear, rewrite your plan as necessary or for an individual's benefit. Pin up customised copies at your home, place of study, or place of work. Encourage friends to carry theirs with them at all times and don't be shy of gently performing 'spot-checks' or 'tests' of their understanding.

Emergency drills

Encourage family members and friends to test you with an emergency drill from time to time. Pick an emergency 'keyword' they can surprise you with, perhaps by phone. Go through the motions as if you were reacting severely while alone.

Is your inhaler or adrenaline easily accessible and where it should be? Is your adrenaline within its expiry date? Is your mobile phone switched on, fully charged and functional? Do you know the exact address and postcode of your location? The procedure is useful in highlighting potential problem points you may need to address.

Although it's usually advisable to call emergency services or possibly your doctor if you live in a remote area. When you experience anaphylaxis, there may be some circumstances where someone may need to take you to hospital for or following treatment. It's worth familiarising yourself with the route in your area, and consider some 'dummy runs' with your partner or family members in the car.

Reactions and children

Much of the advice about serious reactions given in the previous pages can be adapted and applied equally to children.

When it comes to reaction management and your child, it is

vital you take your physician's advice on treatment. If your child is at risk of a severe reaction, you should work out an emergency plan with your doctor, especially if he or she is too young or light to be prescribed adrenaline.

If your child has experienced mild reactions in the past, and you recognise a mild reaction in him, a dose of antihistamine syrup suitable for his age and size is usually recommended. Mild reactions may include little more than light nettle rash, redness and itchiness of the skin, and with irritation around the mouth. However, keep your child under extremely close observation for at least a day for any more worrying signs developing.

Anaphylaxis in babies and very young children is not common, but it is important to realise that skin symptoms such as those mentioned above can often be the first signs that a more serious reaction is about to develop or is already under way. In fact, they are present in around 90% of all dangerous anaphylactic reactions. Here are some possible signs of a severe allergic reaction in your child to watch out for:

1. More extensive rashes, flushing/redness and itchiness of the skin, especially around the mouth, head, hands and feet.

2. Nasal congestion, runny nose or streaming eyes.

3. Any breathing distress such as shortness of breath, or wheezing. These are usually the most worrying reactions in a child.

4. Abdominal distress or pain, if vomiting and diarrhoea occurs the reaction is even more severe.

5. Increased or irregular heartbeat.

6. Anxiety, light-headedness, 'floppiness', the more noticeable it is, the more severe the reaction.

If these more major symptoms are present or you have any doubt about whether the reaction is an anaphylactic one or not, you must act fast on your emergency plan. If your child has been prescribed adrenaline for this event, now is the time to use it. Do not delay, as outcomes are better when adrenaline is administered promptly.

However, if you are certain that there are no abdominal, respiratory or cardiovascular symptoms it is usually not recommended to use it. As always, this is something you should speak to your healthcare provider about in advance. If you are unsure, the advice is usually to use adrenaline as instructed.

Most of the advice given earlier in the chapter about administering adrenaline to adults will also apply to children.

If your child is old enough to carry and administer his own adrenaline, he will need to be taught how to recognise a reaction, and how to inject himself. Again, the auto-injector manufacturers can offer advice and trainer pens, and your nurse and doctor can help too. You will find that most children are easily able to understand the instructions and can be responsible with their own medicine.

Asthma relievers, if your child normally uses them, can be used too, of course.

When you call emergency services, stay calm and give clear instructions and information.

Follow up actions depend on what you have decided with your doctor, and the circumstances of the reaction. If your child is conscious and able to swallow safely, antihistamine medication may usually be safely given. Usually, the advice will include to try to keep your child calm and to avoid trying to make the child vomit. Put your child in a position where breathing is made more easy, and loosen any tight clothing. It is worth learning the

CPR (cardio-pulmonary resuscitation) technique because in the rare instance that your child's heart stops or if he or she stops breathing, you will have to administer it.

When they arrive, emergency services will probably be able to administer a first or second dose of adrenaline if it is needed, and your child may be taken to hospital for further treatments and kept in for observation for up to 24 hours.

Before you leave, if you need it, ask medics for as much information as possible on allergy avoidance. If you do not know what the trigger was, ask for a referral letter to an allergy assessment clinic, or for a letter for your doctor. It is vital to understand the cause.

Ask whether your child is old enough to carry adrenaline. If he or she is prescribed it, make sure you and your child understands, if he is old enough how to use it. This is important for future days, weeks and months, but also for the near future, in case a late phase reaction occurs. You should keep a close eye on your child for this.

Your child's school will also need to be informed that he will be carrying adrenaline, and, as in the case of adults, as described earlier, action plans and emergency drills can be useful for your child. There's more information in Chapter 5, Practical Issues.

Adrenaline Q&A

Q: I'm nervous about adrenaline. Are there any risks involved?

A: When used according to the instructions and in the doses recommended by your allergist or doctor, adrenaline is a safe drug. It's only potentially unsafe for those with heart conditions or when accidentally injected into a vein rather than the thigh muscle. If you are hesitant about any aspect of your allergy medication, speak to your doctor or allergist.

Q: What if I forget my adrenaline?

A: Return home to fetch it. Consider having spare adrenaline
    pens or ampoules and syringes at various sites, such as your
    home, school and office.

Q: What if I suffer a reaction and don't have my adrenaline?

A: Call emergency services at once. Alert someone nearby. If
    you find yourself very near a pharmacy or doctor, try to seek
    help there. Avoid running or rushing about, though, as this can
    speed up the reaction.

Q: I'm pregnant. Can I use anti-allergy medication safely?

A: Anaphylactic incidents in mothers-to-be are rare. When they
    occur, your unborn child may be partly protected by the
    placenta, which produces a defensive, deactivating chemical
    against histamine. While using adrenaline carries a small risk
    to the unborn child, normal recommendations are that your
    well being must take priority. Seek specialist advice about
    your medication as soon as you discover you are expecting.

Which medication – a summary

It is impossible to give a definitive full proof guide, because
reactions can vary so much from person to person, depending on
so many factors. However, good general rules to keep in mind
are:

1. If there are only mild reactions in the mouth, an itchy throat,
    sneezing, a light rash etc, and there are no signs of wheezing,
    shortness of breath, faint feeling or dangerous swelling then
    use antihistamines, and remain on guard for a worsening of
    symptoms.

2. If there is some very light wheezing in addition to the above
    symptoms then use antihistamines and an inhaler, and remain
    on guard for a worsening of symptoms.

3. If there is any systemic itching and rashes, more severe
    wheezing or shortness of breath, faint feeling, sudden acute
    feeling of sickness, or dangerous swelling, especially around
    the mouth and throat then use adrenaline at once.

4. If in doubt then use adrenaline at once.

Chapter 4

Food Sense

The key to managing food allergies is to avoid those trigger food or foods which tests reveal you or your child are allergic to. This is especially important for those at risk of very severe reactions.

Some sufferers may be advised to not only avoid their trigger foods, but also foods which are related to those foods.

Usually, anyone with a serious allergy to one tree nut or peanut, will be advised to avoid all types of nut, because of the high risk of cross reactions or cross contamination.

Likewise, anyone with a serious allergy to any type of seafood, such as fish, molluscs or shellfish, will usually be advised to avoid all others, and anyone with a serious allergy to one animal milk, will usually be advised to avoid all other milks as well.

Appendix 3 on Food Families may help you consider what other foods you may react to or may need to avoid. However, it's important that you only avoid foods you are certain you react to or foods which your doctor or allergist feels you ought to be cautious about. If you have been safely eating foods which are related to your trigger foods, with no reactions and you are certain that there is no risk of cross contamination, there is usually no reason for you to stop eating them. Do not avoid many types or classes of food unnecessarily or without professional advice, especially in the case of children. There is a risk of malnutrition and associated complications if diets become too restricted. Chapter 7 on Nutrition and Health can advise further.

Labelling

With thousands of prepared foods now in our supermarkets, each containing as many as several dozen ingredients, the food sensitive customer has to negotiate a potential allergic minefield.

Food labelling in developing countries lags behind that in Europe, North America and Australia, where strict regulations are in place, but the situation is under way and improved labelling practices, together with wider awareness of food sensitivities, means the outlook is brightening.

Labels on pre-packaged products can sometimes contain vast amounts of information, much of which many people ignore, or misunderstand, or both. As a food allergy sufferer, you cannot afford to do either.

Products may contain the name of the food, nutritional data such as protein, fat and carbohydrate content, energy value, and important dates, such as those of manufacture and of recommended use-by expiry dates. There may also be country of origin and any specific health claims or advice which have been approved.

Elsewhere in the world, the situation varies. In India, according to new Ministry of Health and Family Welfare guidelines, ingredients will also have to be stated in descending order of weight or volume. This sounds positive, but as far as the food allergy sufferer is concerned, there may remain some possible problems.

One proposed guideline states that 'If an ingredient is a combination of two or more ingredients (for example in a namkeen mixture) the compound ingredient has to be declared in the list accompanied by a list of its ingredients. This is not required if the compound ingredient is not a food additive and is less than 5% of the food.'

So if a compound ingredient forms less than 5% and is not a food additive, its ingredients do not have to be declared. Unless you can be certain by calling the manufacturer and checking, for example, you should be wary of such foods.

Another guideline reads 'Flavoring agents don't have to be disclosed'. As flavor can be derived from all sorts of plant and animal products, again this could mean potential allergens are not declared.

Without precise labelling of allergens, many consider the best option to be to avoid all processed and pre-packaged foods, especially in the case of extremely serious allergies.

Where labelling is thorough and detailed, you must not only read them the first time you buy the product, but keep checking every time you buy it in the future, as product ingredients and manufacturing can change with no warning.

Also if you travel abroad and find a familiar product, remember that local ingredients may be different. Always check.

'May contain...'

So-called defensive labelling, that is, 'may contain traces of nuts', for example, is used by some international manufacturers for two reasons: to warn the public that a particular allergen, although not intentionally added, might have accidentally contaminated the product or its ingredients somewhere along the growing, harvesting, transporting or manufacturing line; and also to disclaim any liability in the event of a customer suffering a severe reaction because of a rogue allergen.

This declaration is not a legal requirement anywhere, but increasingly it seems food producers are using it both when necessary and also perhaps when unnecessary. Many consumers are dismayed by this, arguing that it can be confusing to sufferers left unable to gauge the degree of risk of contamination because the message is vague and non specific. Too much 'may contain' labelling also restricts food choices for people with food allergies.

Nevertheless, cases of nut traces (and other allergens) turning up in foods carrying 'may contain' warnings are far from unknown, so you must always take notice of 'may contain' messages if you have a serious allergy.

Unfortunately mistakes can be made, and there are a lot of cases, on record of serious errors being made with food labels even with major international food producers. You should always have your medication with you to protect youself against accidental exposure.

Other labelling information

Alternative means of conveying allergy information can be used.

Some products carry handy 'allergy advice' sections, summarising key information. Look out too for signs such as 'suitable for vegetarians/vegans' which denote that products are free from fish, crustaceans, molluscs and meat, and in the case of vegan, from egg, dairy and honey too.

Calling customer helplines can help answer questions; staff are now getting more and more used to handling allergy queries. You can also write to manufacturers to enquire about their allergy policy. Be specific. The more we question companies in this way, the more allergy aware they will become and the likelier they will implement improvements. Many larger firms can supply list of guaranteed risk-free foods, others can confirm they operate factories free from certain allergies.

Finally, bear in mind that products in ethnic stores and delicatessens, sourced from outside the country, may be imported carrying insufficient, mistranslated or otherwise unclear labelling, perhaps not in a language you can read. Nuts, for instance, can be described in obscurely coded terms, such as 'fruits in shell'. Always steer clear from these products unless you can be certain they are safe.

Shopping

The bad news is shopping with a food allergy is frustrating and time consuming. The good news is the situation is ever improving.

The biggest development worldwide comes in the 'free-from' food market worldwide. Many manufacturers are specialising in extremely niche ranges which are guaranteed nut-free, wheat-free, dairy-free and soy-free, for example, especially for people with food sensitivities. Increasingly, these foods are being imported into India, Asia and Africa and stocked at larger supermarkets. The benefits of these is that they are clearly labelled with allergy information.

There are drawbacks to free-from foods, though.

Firstly, they can be costly.

Secondly, they're not always the healthiest of products. Often, they're heavily sweetened, or processed, or they contain a host of additives or unusual ingredients. This is because in trying to produce safe products which are as free from as many allergens as possible, manufacturers often have to cast their nets wider in search of safe and non allergenic ingredients. These ingredients may help reproduce the characteristics of what has been removed, for instance, xanthan gum as a gluten replacement in wheat-free bread or help mimic the effect or taste of one of the major absent allergens in the free from alternative. Additionally, sometimes the processing method demands the use of extra ingredients, such as preservatives or additives, to help prolong shelf life or improve taste.

Thirdly, manufacturers are occasionally guilty of making an inappropriate virtue of their free-from status. Products claiming to be 'allergy friendly' should be treated with the same caution as any other unfamiliar product. A wheat-free product may indeed be friendly to a wheat allergic person, but it may also be hostile to a nut allergic person. No food is ever completely 'allergy friendly', it depends entirely on the sufferer, not the product.

The golden rule remains that carefully read the label of every item that goes into your shopping basket, no matter how familiar, every time you shop. And if you can't guarantee safety, leave it on the shelf.

And with regard to non pre-packed food sold at bakeries and deli counters or food bought from street sellers or market stalls, sadly cross contamination is a real possibility here, simply because of close storage, handling, or through a 'wandering' spoon or knife. Also, meat products may be sliced on machinery also used for cheeses, transferring allergens between the two. By all means enquire of staff, but it is unlikely they will be able to offer the absolute guarantee you may need. It will not be worth the risk if you have a severe allergy.

Tree nuts and peanuts

It's wise to avoid all nuts and their products if you are allergic to any one or more, due to the risk of cross reactions, cross contamination on production lines, or both unless you are certain neither presents a risk.

A reminder: as allergies in this category are potentially so serious, it is vital you read and re-read all labels. Any 'may contain' warnings must be heeded. Typically, the culprits are found in the following foods, although this list cannot be complete.

1. Praline, marzipan, frangipane, farsan and nougat, and some sweets, desserts, biscuits, yoghurts and chocolate products.
2. Some vegetarian products such as nut roasts and vegetable burgers.
3. Some spreads like peanut butters, nutella.
4. Some mixed cereals and cereal bars.
5. Some satays, curries, stir-frys and chillies.
6. Some salads and salad dressings.
7. Unrefined nut oils or vegetable oil blends (refined nut oils are usually safe).
8. Some alcohic liqueurs.

In the case of chocolate and cereal bars, even when there are no nuts listed in the ingredients, and the products are apparently nut-free, there is often the real possibility that the foods have been manufactured on machinery which has processed nut products previously. If this machinery has not been washed thoroughly, nut traces can remain in the production line, and contaminate supposedly nut-free products. It is worth calling manufacturers to ask whether they can guarantee safety.

Tree nuts will be labelled unambiguously, but peanuts occasionally go by the names of groundnuts, monkey nuts, or earth nuts. You should also look out for peanut sprouts which can look like beansprouts and may be used in Chinese dishes.

Because of cross reactivity, some seeds are a risk to people with nut allergies. Pine nuts (actually seeds) can be a hazard, for example, beware of their use in Italian pesto sauce, as well as in other foods in which nuts are often found. Cross reactions with coconut and nutmeg are uncommon, and in those cases the responses are usually milder. Water chestnuts should be safe, though tree chestnuts may not be.

Some gums used as additives are derived from obscure legumes related to peanuts such as locust bean gum, guar gum, gum tragacanth, acacia/arabic gum and tara gum but the threat to peanut allergics is low. Other daals, beans, lentils, peas often pose a problem, though especially chickpeas and lupin.

Fish, crustaceans and molluscs

These three are biologically distinct, so in theory cross reactions should not occur between members of different groups. If you react to members of more than one group, it's likely you have distinct allergies. Cross reactions between members of the same group are common. See appendix 3 for a list of seafood families.

If you react to any seafood, many practitioners suggest you steer clear of all, partly because of the risk of cross contamination at fish counters, markets, or restaurants. That said, tuna allergics can sometimes tolerate canned tuna, as the canning process seems to deactivate some allergens. Do not experiment, though, if you are uncertain. Typical products to avoid or check carefully are:

1. All fish based dishes, such as kedgeree or fish curries.
2. Sauces such as fish sauce, oyster sauce, Worcestershire sauce.
3. Japanese foods such as sushi, sashimi and surimi/crabstick which may contain white fish and shellfish.
4. Fish pâtés and pastes.
5. Salads such as Caesar's salad, tuna Niçoise or shrimp cocktail.

6. Some stocks, soups, processed foods, sauces and ready meals.
7. Any foods fortified with fish oils (ie 'omega 3 rich' foods).

Note that calcium and glucosamine sulphate supplements may be derived from shellfish. Vegetarian and vegan food is seafood free; Jewish (kosher) food products are shellfish free.

Fish may also be used as a fining agent, for instance in wine.

Wheat and related gluten grains

The use of wheat is widespread, partly because of its additional role as a thickener or stabiliser. Products include:

1. Many flours (for example, atta flour, graham flour), breads, rotis, chapattis and baked products, both sweet and savoury.
2. Many cereals.
3. Many pastas, some noodles.
4. Processed meat and fish products like burgers, pies, sausages, pâtés and battered products like fish fingers.
5. Processed vegetarian products like battered vegetables, pâtés, some tinned vegetables and soups.
6. Some processed dairy products, such as cheese spreads, thickened milks and creams.
7. Drinks, including beers (usually made from barley, but sometimes wheat) and instant drinks or malt beverages.
8. Confectionery including some chocolate bars, sweets, chewing gum and liquorice.
9. Stock cubes, some condiments such as soya sauce and blended seasonings.

Ingredients which can be made from wheat include cereal binder, cereal filler or cereal protein. Hyrolyzed or textured vegetable protein (HVP/TVP) may, rarely, also be made using wheat (more commonly soy), although these are less likely to pose a problem as their intense processing destroys some allergens.

Gluten is the dominant protein in wheat, and gliadin, a constituent of gluten is a main wheat allergen. Consequently, other gluten grains like rye, barley, kamut, spelt, triticale are prime candidates for cross reactions. If you are gliadin allergic, foods labelled gluten-free foods should be safe.

It is possible to be allergic to wheat proteins other than gliadin/gluten. Any foods labelled gluten-free are often but not always wheat free, so take care.

Wheat-free products are now more common, though be aware of the danger of cross reactions with other gluten grains such as barley used as wheat substitutes, especially in flours, pastas and breads.

Oats are also gluten grains, but are more removed from other family members, and so cross reactions are less likely. You may be able to tolerate oats if you're allergic to other gluten cereals especially if they are pure oats. Check the ingredients on oat based products carefully to ensure wheat flour has not been added. If your wheat allergy is severe, it is better to avoid oat products due to the risk of cross contamination.

Dairy food

Obvious products here are milk, cheese, paneer, cream, yoghurt, ice cream, curds, ghee and butter.

A few dairy allergics may find they can tolerate UHT, evaporated or condensed milks, and traces of milk found in some ready meals which have undergone a lot of processing. If you have been eating certain products without problem since your milk allergy diagnosis, it is generally considered okay for you to carry on. Always exercise caution, though, and check with your consultant.

Vigilance is necessary, as milk products turn up in an array of foods and these include:

1. Sweet baked products, such as cakes, pancakes and biscuits.
2. Savoury baked goods, such as breads, crisps and crackers.
3 Sweets and confectionery, including most chocolate.
4. Ready meals, processed meats, convenience products.
5. Soups, curries, stews.
6. Dips, spreads, dressings and sauces.
7. Cereals and snack bars.
8. Instant hot drinks and cream liqueurs.
9. Some sweeteners.

Unusual terms denoting milk extracts include casein, (sodium or potassium) caseinate, curds, lactose, lactalbumin, lactoglobulin and whey.

Look for vegan foods and those labelled dairy-free. Soya milk and cheese make good substitutes. Becoming increasingly available, especially as imports are other milks and milk replacement products made from other legumes, grains and nuts such as pea milk, rice milk, oat milk and almond milk.

Cream of tartar and cocoa butter are dairy free.

Eggs

Allergy to egg white is more common than to yolk, but as cross contamination cannot be guaranteed against, and labelling may not be specific, it is safer to steer clear of all egg containing products if you're allergic. Aside from obvious sources such as quiches, omelettes, mayonnaises many prepared foods also contain egg. These include:

1. Egg noodles, fresh pastas and sauces.

2. Many baked goods, such as biscuits, buns, pastries and cakes often as a glaze.
3. Processed and breaded or battered foods.
4. Dressings and sauces (e.g. Hollandaise, tartare).
5. Some desserts and confectionery such as custard, mousse, meringue, crème caramel, some ice creams, marshmallows.

The additive lecithin, although usually soy derived, is very occasionally produced from yolk.

Egg may also sometimes be used as a fining agent, for instance, in wine and soup stocks, and in some prepared coffee drinks.

Unusual terms denoting egg extracts include albumin, apovitellin, globulin, ovomucin, ovalbumin and vitellin

Soy/Soya

Used abundantly in Chinese and Japanese cuisines, soy is widely used as a dairy protein and meat alternative, and its flour as a wheat flour replacement. It is found in many foods, especially prepared foods, and so is tough to avoid. These are a few examples:

1. Most vegan/vegetarian burgers, pies, sausages, pâtés and prepared meals, and many meat equivalents.
2. Soy milks, and 'cheeses'.
3. Many other specialist dietetic products, such as gluten-free foods.
4. Some cakes, biscuits, pastries and confectionery.
5. Fermented soya products, such as soya/shoyu sauce, tofu, tempeh, natto and miso.
6. Some infant food formulas.
7. Any prepared food labelled hydrolyzed or textured vegetable proteins (HVP/TVP – usually soy), vegetable starch or gum (also often soy), soya caseinate, soy lecithin and monosodium glutamate (often a soy processing by-product).

Daal

As a terrific source of protein, especially for vegetarians, daals are very difficult to avoid, even though you may not need to avoid all. However, in prepared foods there is often a risk of cross contamination between all daals and their flours, so if you are highly allergic, you must take extreme care.

Chickpea / chana daal is a major allergen, and is found in besan / gram flour. Chickpeas can be used for any number of snacks and sweetmeats, and savoury dishes such as stews and curries in India, as well as many foods of middle Eastern and Mediterranean origins.

Of the little known allergens, lupin (or lupine) is considered one of the most dangerous, because it can cross react with peanut and other related legumes, including chickpea. Commonly used in France and neighbouring countries in Europe, high protein sweet lupin is becoming popular as a soya replacement, and its flour is used in bakery, pastries, pastas and other catering, fast food products, such as meat, fish or vegetable batters. Sometimes it shows up unexpectedly in cereals, snack bars, and chocolate or carob confectionery. It is safer to avoid lupin if you have a known allergy to any legume.

Sesame and other seeds

Sesame is found in the Mediterranean and Middle Eastern foods houmous, halva and tahini, and widely in Chinese and other Asian cuisines.

Seeds such as sesame, poppy, pumpkin and sunflower which can cross react with each other and with nuts are increasingly used in a variety of products, sometimes unexpectedly.

1. Baked goods, such as speciality breads, burger buns, biscuits, crackers and cakes, often as decoration and any unwrapped or loose bakery products which may be contaminated.

2. Many prepared meals, such as burgers, vegetable burgers, sausages, curries and nut roasts.
3. Cereals and cereal snack bars.
4. Unrefined seed oils such as sesame oil, Chinese stir-fry oils or oils used in salad dressings and spreads (sunflower spread).
5. Spice mixtures, such as gomashio (Japanese sesame salt).

Celery

Found in traditional Waldorf salad (and perhaps other prepared salads), many vegetable stocks or stock cubes, the rice dish jambalaya, in celery spice and other seasonings, in many Italian tomato based pasta sauces and in health tonics such as 'detox' juices.

Corn/maize

Corn allergy is a widespread problem is North America. Obvious sources such as sweetcorn, corn flakes, other cereals and Italian polenta (cornmeal) aside, products to check include:
1. Ready meals, soups and sauces.
2. Ready made desserts and confectionery.
3. Mexican tortilla wraps and chips, tacos and other convenience snacks.
4. Baked goods, especially specialist gluten-free products.
5. Some baking powders.
6. Any label reading vegetable protein, or hydrolyzed or textured vegetable protein (HVP/TVP – occasionally corn derived).
7. Any label reading edible starch, food starch, modified starch, vegetable starch, cereal starch, glucose syrup (all may be corn derived), corn syrup, maltodextrin or dextrose, though the risk is very low in these instances.

Meat

Allergy to meat is rare, and thorough cooking destroys many of its allergens. It is easy to avoid. Cross reactions between egg, chicken and turkey are possible, as they are between beef and milk. Reactions to processed meat products may be due to added milk, soy or wheat as these are all used widely in prepared meals and meat dishes. Foods reliably labelled vegetarian or vegan will be safe.

Tomatoes

Tomatoes are found in many prepared products. Check all pasta sauces, red-coloured pasta, chillies, pizzas, curries, condiments (chutneys, ketchups), baked beans and other tinned foods, concentrates, soups, salads and juices.

In those with OAS related tomato allergy, only raw tomatoes seem to pose a problem, usually the riper the tomato, the worse the reaction.

Mushrooms and fungi

Mushrooms are found in some prepared meals, stir-fries and salads, and in some sauces, flavourings and stock cubes. Cross reactions with related foods such as truffles and mycoprotein made from a form of fungus are possible.

Other vegetables

Reactions to other cooked vegetables are quite uncommon, but if you suffer you will need to scrutinise labelling on all prepared meals, foods and products such as soups and stock cubes.

Raw vegetable juices are increasingly used in juice blends, and of course raw vegetables will be found in prepared salads.

Alcoholic beverages and aperitifs, and health or 'detox' tonics often contain vegetable extracts. Some of these are surprising. In particular members of the daisy family, including artichoke, dandelion, echinacea and milk thistle, are used in many concoctions. Those with weed related OAS which can cross react with daisy family members should take care.

Fruits

Depending on your allergies, and whether or not you only react to the raw fruit, you may need to check items such as fruit salads, jams, chutneys and other condiments, fruit vinegars (and salad dressings), desserts, chocolates and confectionery, cereals and cereal bars, herbal and fruit teas, and even ready meals.

Take especial care with juice blends, as the name of the product may only mention one or two fruits, yet the ingredients may show the presence of others.

The same goes for spirits, many of which are flavoured with fruits, such as Calvados (apple) and Cointreau (orange).

Those with apple allergy should check for the carbohydrate pectin, derived from apples (or sometimes orange), and used as a setting agent, for instance in jams, in which trace allergens might be found. Apple juices and sometimes other fruit juices are also used as sweeteners, often in sugar free products, dairy-free milks and sometimes products such as soups.

For those with fruit allergies related to OAS, most of these are unlikely to pose problems; only the raw fruits and freshly squeezed fruit juices are of concern. Usually, organic, freshly picked or under ripe fruit may be slightly less reactive.

The allergenic proteins responsible for mild oral reactions tend to be destroyed by pasteurisation and processing so juices made from concentrates or stored in cartons outside the chiller cabinet will probably be safe. Similarly, you should be okay with tinned fruit if you have OAS.

Herbs and spices

Spice allergies to mustard and garlic, for example, tend to be more serious than herb allergies to foods such as coriander. As well as prepared meals, beware condiments such as chutneys or pickles, spice mixtures, stock cubes, prepared salad dressings, herbal teas and health tonics. Remember, in small amounts, herbs and spices may be hidden on labels under generic terms such as 'flavourings' or 'spice mix', for instance.

Cooking and eating

Preventing reactions by avoiding your food allergens is the cornerstone of good food allergy management. To succeed, you must make sure every bite of food you eat is safe. Sadly, as you may already know from experience, this is a formidable task.

Pre-Packaged foods

Ideally, any pre-packed or prepared foods or meals to which you may react will remain on supermarket shelves and never accompany you to the checkout. In practice, oversights happen when you're rushed, and potentially troublesome foods can end up in your shopping basket and your kitchen.

So, before you use any foods in your larder, recheck labels. It takes seconds, and could spare you a reaction. Besides, if a partner or flatmate has done your shopping, you may be examining a product for the first time.

Many foods especially 'bumper' boxes or multi-packs come in extra layers of wrapping, so once you've read outer labelling, ensure you read labels on the individual items inside too. There have been cases where external and internal details have not matched. If you ever find a discrepancy, report it to the manufacturer.

Also, scrutinise the food itself. Does it look like the product described on the label? Very rarely packaging errors occur when products end up carrying the wrong sleeves or labelling information.

Cooking

Some people with very severe food allergies cook all their food from fresh ingredients. The main advantages of home cooking are that you can control what goes into your meals and be confident of those meals being safe and wholesome.

Cooking for yourself is also grounding and relaxing, can make you more 'food aware', and cultivates a healthier relationship with food where you look upon it as something to be enjoyed and savoured, not as a potential enemy. From a health perspective, freshly prepared meals based on unprocessed ingredients are likely to provide better nutrition. It can be more time consuming, but to compensate you'll need to devote less time to reading labels.

There are many cookbooks in the US and UK markets aimed at people on restricted diets such as dairy-free, wheat-free, egg-free, corn-free and more. The internet is a good means of tracking down titles; try searching for 'allergy eating' or 'cooking egg-free', for example, Antoinette Savill, Barbara Cousins, Michelle Berriedale-Johnson and Rita Greer are some writers to look out for and there are some books mentioned in the 'Useful Resources' section too. It may be worth endeavouring to find a book devoted to your specific allergy, rather than an 'all-purpose' cookbook which excludes foods to which you may not react. Vegetarian and vegan books are also filled with imaginative ideas.

Denaturing food

Cooking some foods and thereby breaking down their trigger proteins, can make them safe for some people.

Those more likely to benefit are OAS sufferers. Cooking the fruits, vegetables and herbs implicated in OAS usually makes them safe although be aware this is far less likely if you experience reactions to raw foods which are not connected to pollen allergy.

The more fibrous a fruit or vegetable is, the more cooking it is likely to need to thoroughly deactivate its allergens. This does not mean, though, that you should cook all vegetables into a pulp, but that some cautious experimentation with cooking times is advised to establish tolerance thresholds. Boiling, steaming, microwaving and roasting are all effective but flash or stir-frying, although very hot, may not denature all allergens if cooking times are short.

Peeling can sometimes make a fruit safe or less reactive. Those with mild apple allergies related to hay fever sometimes find this, because many apple allergens are concentrated under the skin.

However, food preparation itself is not without minor hazards. It is often advisable to ask someone to peel vegetables for you or to wear cooking gloves or a face mask. Closely handling foods to which you react during peeling, slicing or chopping them, for instance, is likely to trigger rashes on your hands, aggravate your eyes and nose and possibly make you wheezy if you inhale vapours. Cooking vapours generally from boiling or frying can also trigger symptoms of wheezing.

Cooking will certainly not denature all allergens. Many still react to some spices, and to celery, for instance. Cooking will have little or no beneficial effect on seeds and nuts, which are best avoided if you react to them.

As always, it is better not to experiment, at least not without the advice and supervision of your allergist or doctor.

Latex-food cross reactions

The allergenic proteins found in tropical fruits and other foods implicated in cross reactions with latex allergy are tougher than those found in fruit and vegetables connected to pollen sensitivities. More intense and prolonged cooking is likely to be required to remove or reduce the possibility of a reaction, although in many cases heat will have no effect.

Cooked potato, for example, is usually well tolerated, as is cooked banana. The allergens in chestnut and avocado are resistant to heat treatment. However, everyone reacts differently, so exercise caution unless you are certain a food is safely prepared in a certain way and again never experiment with foods.

Other foods

In general, those reacting to the major allergenic foods need to avoid all forms of their triggers.

It is impossible to cover all permutations, but there can be exceptions. Cooking can alter the allergenicity of both fish and egg, both for the better and worse, depending on the individual.

If you have been consuming a particular food or product cooked or processed in a certain way with no problem since your diagnosis, then it is generally considered safe to assume you may carry on doing so. Beware, though, of complacency, should you react to raw egg but not cooked, for instance, an omelette prepared to quickly can have consequences.

Replacement ingredients

Finding replacements for ingredients you use regularly can be difficult at first, but specialist allergy cook books can provide some ideas. Here are some suggestions:

Milk: Try natural coconut milk in sweet recipes, or in hot drinks or on cereal try any of the range of other alternative 'milks' now widely available, including soya, oat, almond, hazelnut and potato.

Cheese: Tofu, soya 'cheeses'.

Cream: Creamed coconut or other nuts pasted and blended with warm water and maybe honey.

Yoghurt: Soya yoghurts or desserts; for dressings or dips, experiment with plain mayonnaise.

Wheat flour: For baking, try a mix of other flours such as rice, buckwheat and potato combined with either guar or xanthan gums to prevent crumbling. For thickening cornstarch, tapioca or arrowroot are good.

Pasta: Rice noodles, buckwheat noodles (soba) or corn pasta.

Cereal grains: Try buckwheat (not a true wheat), quinoa, amaranth, millet.

Egg: For glazing, try a honey or sugar solution, or gelatine (also a useful setting agent); for binding, try pureed banana or apple, tofu or a soya dessert; for leavening, use baking powder and some liquid.

Nuts and seeds: As a snack, popcorn or other popped grains; fried croutons to add 'crunch' to salads.

Tips for cooking and eating at home

Most people adapt easily to the changes required by a diagnosis of food allergy, and quickly establish workable routines, so will you. Here are some tips which may help:

1. Wash (or peel) all fresh produce that may have come into contact with other people or foods as allergen traces can spread easily.
2. Get organised with menu planning. It helps to dictate efficient weekly shopping and avoid last minute what-to-cook dilemmas.
3. Cook safe sauces and soups and other staples in large quantities, and freeze batches, so that you always have allergy safe home cooked meals available when you come home tired and hungry, or to feed allergic family members, all at short notice.
4. Have safe ready-to-eat snacks in cupboards too, in case you really can't wait.
5. Never reuse oils in which you've previously cooked unsafe foods.
6. Guard against absent minded sampling of food if you're cooking for family members who don't share your allergy – chewing a piece of gum can help.
7. In large households, take care with cross contamination like traces of dairy spreads in the jam jar, wheat toast crumbs in the butter tray and encourage everyone to use separate items of cutlery for each food.
8. Have separate utensils for cooking allergen safe and non allergen safe foods, and closely examine them to ensure they're spotless before use.
9. If you try new foods, check the food families they or their ingredients belong to first, so you can identify any potential cross reactors. Only ever do so when you are not alone, have your medication, and are close to a phone and preferably try them in the morning or early afternoon when you're more likely to be alert to any possible reaction and less likely to have had alcohol.
10. Store allergic foods separately in plastic containers in the fridge for instance and where they can't contaminate or

be contaminated by other foods such as by a leaking milk carton.

11. Aim to keep a clean, tidy, hygienic kitchen, as good kitchen management will guard against slip-ups. To keep kitchen hygienic wash cupboards, refrigerators and worktops regularly.

12. In the case of serious allergies within a large household, consider imposing a total ban on the food in question as do most families with a nut allergic member and ensure everyone, visitors included, understand the rule.

Eating out

Most serious food allergic reactions occur away from the home and are caused by food prepared by others.

Yet eating out is probably an important part of your social life and you should not deny yourself this pleasure, instead, make plans and take every precaution possible to ensure your safety and enjoyment.

Where to eat

Choose restaurants whose cuisines are unlikely to trouble you. Asian restaurants like Thai, Chinese, Malaysian are good choices for wheat and dairy allergics, for example, but not good for fish or nut allergics. Ask fellow allergy sufferers for recommendations. Share your problem with friends and colleagues, avoiding a particular restaurant is not awkward if everyone knows of your condition.

Call ahead if you plan to eat at a restaurant to ask whether you can be catered for. If your condition is life threatening, emphasise it in clear terms. Be direct with questioning. Be prepared for the person taking your call to put you on hold to check with chefs. If ultimately they sound doubtful, don't book the table.

If you intend dining at a high profile or high street restaurant, it's worth searching its website or calling its customer services helpline to find out its policy on food allergy. Some are excellent in this respect, and can let you know which meals, whose ingredients are often standardised, might be safe.

Eating or drinking at an independent cafe, takeaway outlet or bar can be riskier, because food production is unlikely to be as controlled and ingredient lists may not be available.

Be aware that you can be exposed to allergens in surprising ways like foamed eggs are occasionally used as toppings on coffee or other bar drinks and foods at self-service areas can easily be cross contaminated by wandering cutlery. If the chef has used latex gloves in preparing food, traces of milk proteins which are used in latex glove manufacture can transfer to food and trigger a reaction in dairy allergics.

Ordering

When you arrive at a restaurant where you haven't pre-booked a table, make sure you inform a member of staff immediately about your allergy. Ask if they can check whether there are safe foods available. Don't be shy of explaining the precise consequences of contamination or errors. Ensure your conversation is witnessed by members of your party. If you are not confident the seriousness of your condition is appreciated, don't eat there.

Read menus carefully. Never let hunger or impatience get the better of judgement. Ask waiting staff to clarify ambiguities and specify safe meals possibly recommended by the chefs. If you can speak to a chef, so much the better; you'll be able to better gauge their degree of confidence in the meal they're serving you.

Don't be shy of questioning staff as they are now accustomed to hearing specific dietary needs and can be increasingly relied upon to convey those needs accurately to kitchen staff.

1. Is the chef 100% certain of all the ingredients he uses in his recipe?
2. Might a food be cooked in oil previously used to cook a risk food, such as fish?
3. Are separate utensils, chopping boards and knives used to prepare different foods?
4. What are the ingredients of the salad dressings?
5. Have the 'safe' desserts been stored well away from the nut containing desserts?

Listen carefully to the replies given. Do this even in restaurants in which you've previously dined and have come to know you. Never become complacent. Suppliers, ingredients, chefs, recipes and menus all change. Always check, every time.

OAS sufferers are better off ordering cooked food, which ensures many allergens have been denatured by heat. Some latex food allergy sufferers may be able to get away with a similar tactic, but the most sensitive needs to take greater care because even the use of latex gloves in the kitchen can leave rubber traces on food to which you may react. Note too that potentially cross reacting enzymic fruits such as mango, pineapple, papaya/pawpaw and kiwi are sometimes used by cooks to tenderise meat.

Understandably, there will be times when you may not want to go through all this. A bit depressing, perhaps, but in this instance plain food is often safest like meat and vegetables. Soups, stews, pies and other dishes where ingredients are disguised or can lie hidden within and undetected are best avoided.

Precautions

Your fellow diners should know about your allergy and about the consequences of you consuming your trigger allergens. Ensure someone has a copy of your emergency procedure (see pg. 33-34) and knows where your medication is kept.

When your food arrives, use your eyes and nose. Does it look and smell as if it is free from your trigger? Ask someone to taste it if you need to, and start off cautiously. Send anything you're suspicious of back. Never pick allergens out of food you are served especially not nut toppings off desserts. Re confirm with waiting staff that your meal is safe in busy restaurants, with many clients to attend to, instructions can be forgotten and mistakes made.

And finally...

Make a point at the end of the meal of thanking staff for catering for you. It will encourage them to become more allergy aware. Further, spread the word and report excellent establishments to other sufferers, and relevant organisations.

Visiting friends

Being invited to dinner and having to inform your hosts of your condition can feel awkward, but you must impress upon them the seriousness of your condition if this is the case. Ease your discomfort by offering to help with the preparations and cooking, or to bring your own safe ingredients or dishes.

Buffets and parties are more problematic, as food arrangements here can be more confusing. Be wary of cross contamination issues, and guard against absent minded nibbling while you're busy socialising. Cocktail snacks like sushi and Chinese bites often have hidden egg and nut.

During national holidays or other festivities, there will be more food around, possibly alcohol, and in the buzz of celebration it is easy for hosts and sufferers alike to forget about allergies. Always be on your guard.

Chapter 5

Practical Issues

Although becoming 'food sensible' is an important skill to acquire in order to effectively manage your allergy, it's inevitable that other aspects of your life will need attention too.

Personal hygiene

Every day we wash, scrub, cleanse, moisturise, deodorise, condition and colour parts of our body with a boggling selection of gels, soaps, sprays, creams, pastes, oils, powders, scents and dyes but what about the safety of the ingredients in these potions?

Cosmetics are big business. In the fierce battle for consumer appeal, beauty and grooming companies are now placing greater emphasis on natural products, a trend which has resulted in more grains, fruits and other botanicals finding their way into toiletries, many of them in unadulterated states, and therefore potentially more allergenic.

So what's the risk? One might think small. Personal care products are not meant for consumption and, barring lipsticks, toothpastes and mouth washes, are not used orally.

However, when you consider that shower gel can get into eyes, bath oils and scents may be inhaled, and around 60% of the make-up, deodorants and creams we apply to our bodies is absorbed through the skin into the bloodstream, the picture becomes more worrying.

Product labelling

In an ideal world ingredients should be listed on personal care products either on the container, or the packaging but they aren't always. With cosmetics which are small and difficult to label clearly, their ingredients should be displayed close to the item's point of sale or available on a leaflet. Ask for assistance from a sales assistant. If you are highly allergic, avoid products which are insufficiently labelled or not labelled at all.

Even when there are detailed ingredients, three issues remain awkward for the consumer, that is, botanicals are often in Latin not English (see list below); the names may refer to any part of the plant like flesh, seed, shell, bark or leaf and it might not always be clear what has been used; and the widespread use of the word 'parfum' (perfume), as a general term for any combination of fragrances (which can trigger allergies in themselves).

Nut derivatives are sometimes used. Peanut goes by the name arachis hypogea and peanut oil by arachis oil and both can crop up in products such as soaps, make-up and emollients. It is safer to avoid nut containing cosmetics if your family has allergies. The same applies, clearly, if you are already sensitised, although only traces of allergen are likely to be present in the case of nut oils, and any reaction will probably be mild and localised. Almond milk (sometimes called badam) is often used in soaps and creams.

Fruit kernels are sometimes used too, and these have the potential to cross react with nuts especially apricot or peach kernels and almonds, which belong to the same family, the rose stone or plum family, or prunus in Latin.

Grains and nuts tend to crop up in products of a thicker consistency, such as gels, creams and exfoliating washes, and fruits are often found in liquid shower gels and shampoos, for instance, but unexpected ingredients are more widespread in cosmetics than in foods, such as deodorants containing wheat protein, aftershaves containing sesame, and many more strange examples.

If you ever see the notation [+/- ...] this indicates that the ingredient(s) listed in square brackets may or may not be present, the cosmetic equivalent of a 'may contain' warning.

Latin names of food allergens in cosmetics

Here is a useful reference list:

Almond – prunus [amygdalus] dulcis/amara/sativa
Apple – malus domestica/pyrus malus
Apricot – prunus armeniaca
Avocado – persea gratissima/americana
Banana – musa sapientum
Barley – hordeum/hordeum vulgare
Brazil nut – bertholletia excelsa
Cashew – anacardium occidentale
Celery/celeriac – apium graveolens
Chestnut – castanea sativa/sylva
Chickpea – cicer arietinum
Coconut – cocus nucifera
Corn – zea mays
Egg – ovum
Fish/fish oil – pisces/piscum iecur
Hazelnut – corylus rostrata/avellana
Kiwi fruit – actinidia chinensis
Lupin – lupinus albus/luteus

Macadamia nut – macadamia ternifolia
Milk – lac
Oat – avena sativa
Peach – prunus persica
Peanut – arachis/arachis hypogea
Pistachio – pistacia vera
Rice – oryza/oryza sativa
Sesame – sesamum indicum
Soya – glycine max/soja
Sunflower – helianthus annuus
Walnut – juglans regia/nigra
Wheat – triticum/triticum vulgare

Other reactions to cosmetics

Contact dermatitis, characterised by red itchy patches of skin is
the most common reaction. It is usually non-allergic and triggered
by an irritant such as an abrasive or a detergent. The reaction is
delayed not immediate, localised to the site of application, and
usually caused by repeated exposure to the cosmetic, rather than
one-off use. Eczema sufferers and light skinned people are more
susceptible, but irritant contact dermatitis can effect anybody.

Genuine allergic contact dermatitis is less common. It is often
caused by one or more of the many thousand fragrances found
in bodycare products, but also by preservatives, UV filters and
emulsifiers. Unlike irritant contact dermatitis, allergic contact
dermatitis can spread beyond the site of application. Patch testing
by a dermatologist can help identify culprits. Around 2% of the
population may be allergic to at least one cosmetic ingredient; and
people prone to other allergies, including food allergies are more
susceptible.

Immediate urticarial rashes are occasionally reported too, as are
'burns' to assorted substances. Tragically, one or two anaphylactic

deaths have occurred due to exposure to chemical hair dyes. Also you should always avoid any henna products which may not be pure and trustworthy, as adulterated henna can cause serious burns and allergies in some individuals.

Cosmetic safety

Read all labels on products, for both ingredients and instructions, and perform a patch test if recommended.

Some botanical extracts in cosmetics have the potential to cross react with allergens to which you are already sensitised.

Check the safety of products used by your hairdresser, beautician or even massage therapist. If you are severely reactive, avoid bathing or grooming when alone at home, or behind a locked door.

If dermatitis is a concern, avoid certain products for short periods to see whether symptoms ease. Don't stick to favourites, rotate safe products to avoid risking sensitization through continued use. Don't use products on broken skin. Products calling themselves 'hypoallergenic' should be free from fragrances and are less likely to cause reactions, but there are no guarantees. The expression 'dermatologically tested' is largely meaningless.

Domestic issues

Your home should be your safe haven, but when dealing with allergies you must guard against complacency. Although exposure to toiletries perhaps poses the greatest risk of a non-food reaction, there are other sources of potential triggers.

Pets

Animals can cause allergies, particularly the sweat and saliva of cats and dogs while your pet's skin, hair and waste products may trigger asthmatic symptoms. However, as a food allergic individual you should perhaps be more concerned with what you feed your pet.

Pet food can contain key allergens. Ingredients may be declared on the label. Dog food may have cereal grains and milk; cat food often contains fish, crustaceans, molluscs and occasionally grains; bird food may have seeds and cereals as well as milk and egg derivatives; and fish food might contain fish, crustacean, molluscan, cereal and egg derivatives.

Handling food may trigger reactions if you're sensitively allergic. Wear gloves, and take care with opening tins and packets. Keep all pet bowls and cutlery used to dispense petfood separate from domestic crockery. Dogs are messy eaters, and their food can travel across floors and be deposited on furniture only to end up on hands and be transferred to the mouth. So, its better to clean up regularly and keep alert. You may need to discourage your affectionate pet from licking you enthusiastically after a feed too. If you can house or feed your pet outside the home, for instance in a designated garden or shed area, so much the better. In all cases, never allow your pets into your bedroom, which should be your allergy free haven.

Household cleaning

Products such as polishes, air fresheners, washing liquids and powders, bleaches and detergents sometimes contain plant extracts, but any reactions you experience to them are likely to be chemical sensitivities not allergies.

Some of these products, and others such as aromatic candles, will also have one or more potentially allergenic fragrances, of the sort used in cosmetic products. Ingredients are rarely provided, so call manufacturers, and see your doctor if you experience symptoms.

Gloves and masks help minimise contact while cleaning, but it's a good idea generally to try to reduce your chemical exposures inside the home, as they can challenge the body and the immune system; why not throw open the windows instead of using air freshener, or try damp clothes not furniture sprays to wipe surfaces?

Keeping dust mites and cockroaches to a minimum may also help your allergies, especially if you experience cross reactions to shellfish.

Here are some tips to beat dust mites:

1. Wash bedding, pillows and duvets in hot water at 60 degrees and consider using protective coverings over mattresses and pillows.

2. Keep the home and bedroom well ventilated to reduce humidity.

3. Vacuum regularly with a high quality cleaner.

4. Use a damp duster on all surfaces.

5. Have as few carpets as possible and choose rugs which can be washed regularly.

6. Keep curtains and soft furnishings to a minimum.

7. Keep pets out of the bedroom.

8. Expose mattresses, rugs, carpets and bedding to strong direct sunlight for several hours as this can kill mites.

Here are some to beat cockroaches:

1. Tackle them with the best and safest insecticides you can use.

2. Keep all foods safely away in sealed containers and cupboards.

3. Close all cracks in floors and walls especially in rooms where food is kept.

4. Avoid dampness in the home.

5. Check regularly for signs of cockroaches, and wash and scrub floors periodically with detergent to keep them free of allergens.

Gardening and Pollens

Asthma or hay fever sufferers are susceptible to pollen, spores, mould and fragrances from the garden, but you can take steps to reduce exposure. Insect pollinated plants, such as most flowers, are safer to hay fever sufferers than wind pollinated plants, such as trees or grasses. Avoid sniffing potently fragranced flowers, though, and ask someone else to mow the lawn. Wear gardening clothes, sunglasses, a hat and gloves to protect yourself from pollen.

Members of the daisy family including chrysanthemums, dahlias, dandelions, marigolds and feverfew can be problematic to all allergy sufferers too. Handling them may cause dermatitic reactions, and they can also cross react with other, commonly eaten members of the daisy family, such as sunflower and camomile. Take care if you have weed pollen sensitivity.

Fertilisers, plant sprays, insecticides and plant foods can trigger chemical and allergic sensitivities, so protect yourself when handling them. Organic gardening products are more likely to contain plant derived materials such as rape seed, soy and sunflower, so be aware of possible cross reactions.

Finally, don't grow any plants which may trigger allergies

in the family. For instance, avoid sweet lupins or perhaps other legumes if there's a risk of your peanut allergic child coming into contact with them playing in the garden.

Avoiding exposure to pollen may help to reduce your food allergies if you have OAS. Here are some tips:

1. Wear wrap around sunglasses to protect eyes.
2. Use nasal sprays which put a barrier between pollen and your nasal lining or try a smear of petroleum jelly around your nostrils.
3. Keep windows closed during peak pollen times such as early morning and early evening.
4. Hang clothes out to dry on low pollen days or during low pollen times and shake them vigorously before you bring them inside.
5. Change your clothes in a room other than the bedroom to avoid spreading pollen where you sleep.
6. Wash your hair after a day out to rinse away pollen.
7. Keep car windows closed and consider installing pollen filters.
8. Wash your pets to rinse off pollen from their coats after they've been outside.
9. Minimise exposure to pollution, as this can make your pollen sensitivity worse.

Your social and personal life

You must take care in places other than food outlets and restaurants.

In bars, and with regard to drinks, provided you're certain of their ingredients, pre-bottled varieties are generally the safest. Take care with any drinks served in glasses which may not have been scrupulously washed. Bar snacks typically nuts are a bigger problem, though, if you're especially sensitive, as allergens can become airborne when other drinkers are consuming them, and this can trigger a reaction. Remember alcohol clouds your judgement, slows your response and may hasten a reaction.

In night clubs, the mix of dancing, loud noise and alcohol is potentially even more distracting, although there are usually fewer bar snacks. Taking recreational drugs in these situations must be avoided, as some especially in club atmospheres can make you paranoid, depressed or panicky, all of which could compromise your safety and lead you to use medication inappropriately.

At the cinema, many people like to eat snacks such as nuts and popcorn, and sometimes the air can get thick with food aromas. If you're highly sensitive to these allergens, ask to be seated in a secluded area. Check seats carefully for discarded food.

If you like to get amidst a large body of people such as at a rock concert it's better to stick to nothing but water. Getting out of a dense crowd swiftly to access emergency treatment could be impossible in such a situation.

Many are increasingly using gyms, both to keep fit, but also as a means of getting out and socialising. If you carry medication or are susceptible to exercise induced anaphylaxis, you must make senior people at the club and any medical staff such as first-aiders or physiotherapists aware of your condition, and always have a training buddy with you. It's worth checking equipment is clean before you use it. Bear in mind that calorific foods such as milk protein drinks, cereal bars and nut snacks are commonly eaten by keep-fit enthusiasts to keep energy levels high, so are likely to be a constant presence.

Finally, it's worth inputting an emergency contact into your mobile phone under ICE (In Case of Emergency): useful should you have an attack, not only while out on your own, but also should you get separated from responsible friends.

Personal relationships

Kissing someone who happens to have been eating nuts or fish that day could be risky for you. Yes, it is embarrassing, but you must ask! If you're shy, try to introduce some light humour but ensure the seriousness of your allergy is understood by your romantic partner.

Food allergic people report constantly how supportive partners can be to their condition, and yours will almost certainly be no exception. If you need them to sacrifice a food from their diet, they surely will.

Another point for dairy allergics: Some condoms are manufactured using a process employing the milk protein casein. Check whether your condoms are vegan friendly.

Your professional life

If you're pondering a career in the catering or food industries, it could prove difficult to protect yourself from allergens, and employers may be reluctant to take you on. Food allergies may make your life difficult in other jobs too such as caring or nursing, or piloting or airline cabin work.

If as a newly diagnosed food allergic you already work with food, gloves and face masks might help, but may prove impractical.

Whatever your job, you must inform your employers of your condition. Large companies will have personnel departments which can prove supportive and perhaps put you in touch with other allergic employees as well as designated first-aid officers, whom you should train in adrenaline administration. Do likewise with close working colleagues, and consider pinning up emergency action plans on noticeboards or in staff canteens.

Student life

When you combine youthful irresponsibility with the freedom of life away from home and the thrill of forging new relationships and friendships, it's perhaps only to be expected that the importance of food allergy prevention tactics may slip down the list of priorities in a young person's mind when they go off to college or university, but the sad truth is that anaphylactic deaths tend to occur in this age group more than any other.

Parents can go a long way to remind their newly grown-up children of their responsibilities to look after themselves. Urge them to take an interest in their condition, join relevant groups, and read widely on the subject. It's also worth pre-emptively 'training' adolescents for the prospect of leaving home: for instance, by encouraging them even as young children to order their own food in restaurants and explain their allergies to chefs and waiting staff, rather than you doing it for them.

If you are a student, it's important you get used to the implications of fending for yourself and take responsibility for carrying your medication at all times. Many colleges and universities can cater well for those on limited diets perhaps by teaming you up with flatmates with similar restrictions in self-catering, or by guaranteeing nut-free meals at least once a day. The sooner you let the establishment know, the more likely they will be able to arrange help for you.

When there, those who need to know of your allergy may include close fellow students and roommates, the college nurse, your new doctor, your hall of residence warden, the catering manager, your tutors and any university first-aiders. Speak to university medical staff about your condition, and the best procedure in the event of an emergency. You may need to adjust your emergency action plan accordingly. Don't forget to give one to friends, tutors and wardens, perhaps with a clear photograph of you attached. Pin some up on visible noticeboards too.

Larger universities may have student allergy support societies. If there isn't one where you're studying, consider setting one up. It's a terrific way of meeting people in the same boat as you and setting up a network of young people always on the lookout for one another.

School life

Very young children may not comprehend fully the implications of their food allergy, so it is important when sending them to nursery or pre-school that their carers fully understand any dietary requirements and medicines to be given to your child in the event of a reaction. Fellow parents may also need to be informed that not to give their children nut containing snacks to take to school, for instance, as many children casually swap and play with food.

You should set up an action plan with your doctor or allergist, clearly summarising what should be done in the event of your child reacting, such as what medication should be given and at what stage, and who to call. Attach a photo of your child to the plan, and distribute it to essential personnel. Storage of medication is also a vital issue, as children may not be old enough to carry it with them. Staff may have to be trained to use adrenaline. All this should be discussed with the school teachers, nurses and governors to ensure everyone is happy and understands the situation.

Supervision is especially important during lunch times. Reassure yourself that there are always enough teachers supervising the children when food is consumed who are aware of your child's allergies. Some schools with a lot of food allergic children segregate them into separate areas, and while this is clearly safer, it can make children feel excluded, so is not to be undertaken lightly.

Teachers should be made aware of the fact that play doughs and paints can contain allergens (like wheat and egg respectively), and outdoor activities can expose children to wild nuts and seeds and plants.

Remember to educate your child fully too. They must be taught which foods are and are not safe for them, that they should not accept food from other children or consume food which has not been specially prepared for them. Give them advice on how to recognise a reaction, and how to tell a teacher or other carer that they are feeling unwell and may be experiencing one. Role play could be useful here. Regularly 'review' their understanding but without alarming them.

All this applies to older children too, although some may be able to carry their own medication with them, and they should be reminded to do so at all times.

Issues surrounding feeling 'different' or marginalised at school can be a concern for children who want to fit in with all their friends. Encourage teachers to not exclude them from activities because of their food allergies, and to keep vigilant in case of bullying or teasing from other children. Sadly, there have been cases in America of children hiding peanuts within a nut allergic child's lunch as a practical joke, simply because a lot of children cannot understand the potential seriousness of food allergy. Again, speaking with other parents can help.

Medicine and healthcare

Unfortunately, a lot of medicines are manufactured using allergenic foods, including wheat, soy, corn and egg. Dairy is used regularly in medicines and tablets (including oral contraceptives), and even sesame or peanut oil crop up occasionally in pharmaceuticals. Many supplements for the joints, such as glucosamine and those containing essential omega oils, may be derived from shellfish and fish respectively.

Every time you are prescribed medication by your doctor remind him of your allergy. When you collect it from the pharmacist, confirm that it is free of your trigger. Read labels and instructions not just for allergens, but also for any possible interactions with your allergy medication. This applies to inhalants, topical creams and any medicines taken orally or internally.

Do the same with over-the-counter medication or supplements. It's always worth enquiring whether allergy free alternatives are available.

Inform and remind all healthcare workers like dentists, chiropodists, physical therapists of your allergy before they treat you.

Wearing personalised medical alert necklets or bracelets is recommended should you be at risk of anaphylaxis or any other condition which may require emergency treatment, either here or abroad.

Vaccinations

Influenza and yellow fever vaccines are cultured on egg, and pose a potential risk to extremely sensitive egg allergics, should trace proteins be present in the vaccine. Speak to your healthcare practitioner to help ascertain the risk and reassure yourself. The current thinking is that the risk is very low, and that rare reactions to vaccines are due to some other factor. Sometimes, vaccination at a hospital with resuscitation equipment at close hand can be arranged.

Holidays and travel

With all the anxiety of living with food allergy, you probably deserve a break more than most. Advance thinking is essential when it comes to getting away from it all. Don't leave matters until the last minute. Plan for all eventualities.

Before you go

Choose destinations sympathetic to your allergies. If you're dairy or wheat allergic, south east Asia may be suitable, whereas Italy, land of pasta, pizza and Parmesan cheese, may not be. If you're soy allergic, the reverse applies. Bear in mind that western nations have very high rates of food sensitivities and are accustomed to dealing with allergies and restricted diets and helping people with them.

If you're nervous about the language barrier, look for holidays in touristy or resort areas, where English will be spoken, or choose a nation whose main language you can speak. Ask your travel agent about hotels catering for those on restricted diets. If you have multiple or severe allergies, self catering may be the better option. An hour or more spent on the internet searching your chosen location, its dishes, restaurants, health food stores, hotels will be well spent.

Acquire translations to common culprits. Consider having some phrases such as 'I am severely allergic to...' or 'Is this product guaranteed free from...?' translated through a reputable translation agency or see the 'Useful Resources' section for helpful websites and manufacturers of translation cards. If you have any other particular medical requirements that may need to be communicated to healthcare workers while abroad, ask your doctor to write a brief summary, which again you could have translated. You may like to do likewise with your emergency action plan, copies of which you can later give to hotel management and your tour representatives or guides.

Pack essential safe supplies such as allergen-free snacks in case you're caught short, say by flight delays, and take cosmetic items such as sun lotion too. The less shopping you have to do in a foreign country, the better. Foreign versions of foods found on supermarket shelves may contain different ingredients and will be made in a different factory, even if the brand is identical, so a safe product at home may not be a safe product away from home.

Ensure you have enough adrenaline (and other medication); obtaining replacements abroad could be difficult. Check with your travel agent and airline that needles and injectors are allowed in the cabin, and arrange a letter from your doctor to produce at security control or check-in. Remember to pack storage cases for your medication: adrenaline can degrade in the heat of the beach, so you need to protect it carefully.

Ensure your travel insurance covers treatment for your allergy. Wearing medical jewellery abroad with your condition clearly stated on it or inside it.

Air travel

An aeroplane mid-flight is one of the last places you would choose to experience a reaction, and many severe allergy sufferers are, understandably, worried about flying.

Speak to your travel agent or, much better, call and deal with the airline directly. Some airlines operate nut-free catering policies, and some do not serve peanuts, but they cannot stop other passengers bringing snacks on board. Some, however, will make an announcement requesting passengers not to consume nuts on board, if you ask. Others, like Singapore Airlines, may decide not to offer nut-free flights. Airborne nut allergens can

trigger reactions, but only mild ones usually. Snacks handed
out with drinks are more of a concern, as this will cause greater
volumes of allergens to circulate and recirculate in the recycled
cabin atmosphere. Nevertheless, the risk remains low. It's worth
taking along some wet wipes to clean seats and fold down trays in
the event of nut traces left behind from an earlier flight.

The most likely cause of a reaction is through consumption.
The best security is to bring your own food.

When you come to fly, let check-in staff and senior members
of cabin crew know of your allergy. The more people you inform,
the more likely your needs will be accommodated.

When you arrive

As soon as is convenient, speak to your representative, hotel
manager and anyone else involved in your care during your
holiday. Give them as much information about your condition
as possible. Discuss the best action in an emergency in different
situations like when you're at the beach, on a day trip, at the hotel.
Learn the correct local ambulance emergency number, such as 911
in America and Canada, and 112 in much of Europe.

Ask about health shops or natural food stores locally either
at the hotel or at tourist information as you will need to stock
up on safe foods. Assistants here are also likely to be more
knowledgeable about restricted diets than those in supermarkets,
and your translations will be handy. Visit them soon so you get to
know them, or can find alternative stockists if they're unsuitable.

Don't put these errands off, the sooner you get them done and
reassure yourself, the longer you can devote to relaxation.

Eating abroad

One of the toughest aspects of holidaying abroad is having to navigate the culinary wonders that tempt your senses as markets and bazaars heady with the intoxicating aromas of street food, for instance, and delicatessen windows displaying magical tasty delights.

The level of care you take depends largely on the severity of your condition. If you do wish to taste local foods or dishes, ask as many questions as you need to, use your translation cards and ensure you have your medication to hand. When eating out, it may be worth dining outside peak lunch or dinner hours, when waiters and chefs will be less harassed and more able to cater for you precisely.

Take care not only with prepared foods, but also unfamiliar raw fruits and vegetables. African, South American and Caribbean countries, in particular, boast a lot of native produce which never reaches these shores, but which may cross react with your particular allergens. If you have latex fruit cross reactions, bear in mind that other tropical fruits, besides those which you know trigger a response, may also be reactive.

Lots of nations or cultures have their own particular food traditions, products and delicacies, and it is impossible to list all potential dangers.

For instance, almonds and almond flour are liberally used in Spain, Portugal and some Latin American countries in pastries, cakes and other baked goods.

Lupin flour is used widely in France, the Mediterranean and Australia.

In Greece, the beans and seeds are consumed as foods and snacks in their own right.

While wheat beers, as well as the usual barley based beers, are common in Germany, Belgium, Netherlands and Luxembourg

Italian mortadella ham will contain pistachio nuts.

As always, you just have to be on your guard.

Chapter 6

Coping Emotionally

The psychological effects of food allergies are barely discussed, and yet the impact on sufferers and loved ones can be huge, something clinicians are only now appreciating. When so much of your life is spent on the practical implications of your condition by carrying medication, monitoring labels, though, it's easy but ultimately unwise to neglect your emotional health.

Coping with diagnosis

Why me? Is it something I did wrong? These are often the first thoughts of sufferers when they receive confirmation of what they've perhaps suspected for a while. Be assured that in no way are you to blame for your allergy. You, or your child, just got unlucky.

You may feel shocked at this 'failure' of your body, and unable to take in the implications of what you've learned, or you may feel vindicated in discovering that your reactions haven't been 'all in the mind'. In those who have been seeking a diagnosis for many months, that relief may be short-lived, the stress of not knowing what was wrong and perhaps trying to convince your doctor that something was amiss may have been lifted, but now it has been replaced with the anxiety of an uncertain future.

Obviously the most desirable response to diagnosis is a positive, combative one, where you decide to arm yourself with knowledge and tackle the illness head on, refusing to let it get the better of you. It's also beneficial to assess your support network and 'rally the troops' – your personal team of partner, spouse, friends and family, who care for you and can help you come to terms with your condition.

That said, some people, through no fault of their own, find the road to this stage a bumpy one.

Self pity

A brief period spent feeling sorry for yourself can do you good. If you're overwhelmed with your diagnosis and its implications, having a short 'shut down' for a few days could be just what you need, and is perfectly normal. Allow yourself time off work or study. When you emerge from the gloom, as you begin to accept your situation, you will probably find yourself ready to do battle with your allergy.

Shock and anger

You may feel resentful of the situation in which you find yourself, and may take your frustration out on loved ones. These feelings are normal, and will usually pass quickly.

Denial and indifference

Consider these attitudes:

1. 'It's only a bit of tingling and wheezing. I'll be okay so long as I don't eat nuts when out with friends anymore.'
2. 'There's no cure and nothing I can do about it. I'll just put

up with the reactions and carry on as normal. I don't really care.'

3. 'I'll be fine. My family and friends will watch out for me.'

Denying a problem, adopting a recklessly care-free stance, passing the onus of responsibility onto loved ones, these are all common initial responses, especially in teenagers.

While they are not so serious as 'stepping stones' to help temporarily diffuse the initial blow of diagnosis, beware the danger of prolonged denial. If you've read this far, it's unlikely you have such an issue, but these attitudes are worth looking out for if you're a parent of youngsters. Parents and medical professionals must ensure, sympathetically but firmly, that young allergic patients are clear on what they can and can't eat, what the risks are, and so on.

Ongoing emotional problems

Some people, especially those with mild or without life threatening conditions, take food allergy completely in their stride. Others experience occasional or chronic psychological problems or hardships, and it is important be aware of these possibilities.

Complacency

This is a sign that denial is creeping back.

Ask yourself the following questions:

1. Have you taken to regularly ignoring food labels?
2. Are you beginning to take risks with unfamiliar foods in restaurants?
3. Do you often catch yourself thinking, 'Just this once won't hurt'?
4. Have you allowed yourself to slip into a 'take it or leave it' attitude towards your medication?

5. Do you increasingly avoid telling people about your condition?
6. Have you stopped visiting your doctor to discuss your allergy?

The more positive responses, the more likely you are to be sliding into perilous territory. A reaction can often act as a wake-up call in such circumstances, but it is preferable to identify lapses and nip them in the bud.

Although it can effect everyone, teenagers, especially boys, are more susceptible. Seeing themselves as young, strong and immortal, having possibly avoided serious reactions for many years thanks to the vigilance of their parents, and wanting to live a normal lifestyle, they are more likely to expose themselves to high risk situations. Sadly, some individuals keep their risk taking from friends and family to protect them from worry, or so as to not send out the message that their allergy is less serious than it actually is.

Shame and stigma

Tragically, many sufferers feel deeply embarrassed, even stigmatised, by their condition; some report feeling like 'freaks' among their non allergic acquaintances. The distorted perception and widespread ignorance of food allergy among the wide population compounds the problem. People may be sceptical, unsympathetic, and may make you feel conspicuously 'different'. Having to speak to chefs before dining, or standing up to colleagues who are pressuring you to join them at a risky restaurant, is tough.

Children, meanwhile, can feel isolated from their school friends. Sadly, non allergic children may tease allergic children, making them feel more isolated and ashamed.

Sufferers can react to this in two ways by either start avoiding social situations and isolating themselves; or by 'going with the flow', ignoring their illness and taking risks. Both are causes for concern.

Depression

Not all people perceive depression as an illness. For some, it's a choice made after finding oneself in tough circumstances. Indeed, a period of mild depressive withdrawal can act protectively. But when this stretches on a long time, the situation becomes serious.

Those at particular risk include those in middle-to-late age, for whom living with a food allergy can have resonant symbolic overtones. If you're older, allergic illness may make you feel doubly fragile at a time when your body might already be showing other signs of failing. This vulnerability can be much more debilitating than the practical implications of suddenly having to avoid a food.

Symptoms of depression include:

1. Indifference, including to pleasurable activities.
2. Lethargy and tiredness.
3. Disordered sleep and rest patterns.
4. Reduced appetite or, oppositely, comfort eating.
5. Low concentration and motivation.
6. Feelings of inadequacy, uselessness, hopelessness.
7. Loss of self-confidence.
8. Overbearing sadness.
9. Irritability and restlessness.

Anxiety and stress

These are common and often severe.

Some anxiety is important. Stress is a helpful trait to keep you alert to possible danger and ready to respond to it. For instance, it is vital you maintain a low, constant level of vigilance to avoid allergens, and be able to promptly respond to an accidental exposure. Don't look upon stress as all bad.

That said, chronic stress can be debilitating, and is a sign of a problem which needs resolving. Parents of food allergic children are known to suffer extreme, relentless anxiety, and the pressure of living under what is perceived to be a constant threat can be too much for adult sufferers too. Stress also compounds asthma and eczema symptoms.

Symptoms of anxiety include:

1. A dry mouth.
2. Cold or hot sweats.
3. Changes in eating habits.
4. Inability to work or concentrate.
5. Sleep disturbance.
6. Sexual disinterest or dysfunction.
7. Obviously untrue negative thoughts.

Fear

A natural response, in both adults and children. Allergy sufferers may fear all manner of things like being surrounded by unknown foods, having to self inject adrenaline, or dying of a severe reaction. Fear can be justified, or it can be disproportionate to the actual threat, but the feelings can be equally intense, either way.

Panic

Adult food allergy sufferers may be more at risk of suffering from panic attacks, possibly triggered by something such as the sudden realisation during a night out at a restaurant that they have forgotten their medication. The symptoms of chest tightness, fighting for air, hyperventilation, dizziness, visual disturbances can be sudden and acutely distressing, and can be similar to a severe allergic reaction which can confuse the sufferer further. People often feel as if they are about to die, which can further perpetuate symptoms into a vicious circle.

Psychological eating disorders

Little research has been done looking at a link between eating disorders and food allergy, but anecdotal evidence appears to show there is one. Studies suggest that those self-diagnosing their allergies demonstrate higher than average levels of anorexia nervosa and bulimia, though it is unclear whether the eating disorders follow on from the 'allergy', or whether claims of allergy are adopted by some women to legitimise their food exclusions. Media coverage of slim personalities who have supposedly overcome sensitivities and lost weight may be partly to blame.

It is also possible that the great care that some genuine food allergic people need to take with their diets may, in vulnerable individuals, gradually slip towards greater suspicion directed towards other foods and their diet in general, followed by hyper-obsessiveness, extreme food exclusions and, consequently, anorexic type behaviour.

Becoming obsessed with your diet or size, being disturbed by minor weight gain, depression, social withdrawal, and excessive exercise are all signs of a problem.

People with food allergies may also be more at risk of psychological food aversions, where they become mistakenly convinced that more and more foods cause food allergy symptoms, when physically this is not the case. An incidence of food poisoning or a mistaken diagnosis from an alternative practitioner can act as the 'trigger' to an aversion. Again, inappropriate dietary restrictions could be a health risk, with malnutrition a real possibility.

Obsessive Compulsive Disorder (OCD)

Although allergic children are less likely to suffer from stress and anxiety, they are more susceptible to OCD. It may be that the hypervigilance demanded by their illness spills into other areas of their lives, promoting wider obsessive behaviour. They may, for instance, insist on repeatedly washing their hands to keep them clean from imaginary food allergens picked up during the course of the day.

Trauma

If you have lived through the ordeal of a severe anaphylactic reaction you may feel devastated by the experience. The shock of the 'near miss', of perhaps coming close to death, can undermine your stability and be emotionally disabling. People who've ticked along for years with perhaps only minor reactions or none at all can feel especially traumatised if an anaphylactic episode has hit them like a bolt from the sky.

Post-traumatic stress disorder (PTSD) is unlikely in those who have suffered anaphylactic reactions, but not impossible. Flashbacks or powerful visualisations such as of your ambulance rush, or emergency treatment being unable to follow simple, day-to-day routine, hypervigilance and obsessiveness, disrupted sleep and nightmares, and violent behaviour all can be symptoms.

Self-help

Although there are plenty of individuals, specialists and groups who can help, you are undoubtedly the most important person involved in your own emotional care.

Knowledge and positivity

Learn about your allergy, and approach your fact finding mission positively; your aim is to eliminate the anxiety which ignorance breeds. Remind yourself too that your condition, despite perhaps being serious, is absolutely manageable.

Statistics can offer great reassurance, for instance, there may be up to thirty-five million people with food allergy in India and yet there are only upto 200 deaths annually from anaphylaxis, as tragic as those cases are. Relatively speaking, the risks are low.

If there is something you do not understand, a niggling query which is bothering you about your allergy, then resolve to find the answer. If this book can't help, ask your healthcare professional, or look for the answer from a reliable online resource or forum.

Also, try to learn from reactions you have, and see the positive aspects of them. Some people who endure an anaphylactic reaction and successfully rescue themselves with adrenaline come to feel empowered by the experience, and reassured in the knowledge that they can manage even the worst of incidents.

Positive thinking also helps your self esteem and self confidence, which may be dented by your allergic status. Be proud not ashamed when you need to tell, say, restaurant staff of your illness, and don't be afraid to put it in no-nonsense terms that you have a life threatening condition. Practise in front of a mirror. Or consider taking assertiveness classes if you feel this is a problem area.

It is the same with children. Here are some tips:

1. Teach allergic children about their allergy, and to not be ashamed of it.

2. Patiently answer any questions they have, and every now and then 'test' them gently on their knowledge of their medication, for instance.

3. Involve them in food preparation so they come to have a healthy relationship with food, so they don't feel alarmed by it or consider it a danger.

4. Always praise them and encourage them to boost their confidence.

5. If your child feels 'different' because of his food allergy, tell him that differences are okay, and that everyone is different like they have different colour skins and eyes, different heights, different strengths and talents and different tastes and needs.

It also helps to educate your close friends and loved ones. Explain to them carefully about the foods that you or your child can and cannot eat. Tell them about your or your child's medication. Show them this book so they too can learn about food allergies. You will feel much more at ease and secure in the knowledge that those close to you understand the issues surrounding food allergies.

Volunteering

Helping yourself by helping others can work wonders. Volunteering gives something back to the allergic community, and will also strengthen your character and prove deeply fulfilling.

There are plenty of ideas which can help both you and others, like:

1. Could you set up a local support group?

2. Could you act as the point of contact for people in your area?

3. Could you organise regular meetings to keep in touch with fellow sufferers and swap tips and information about food and restaurants?

4. Can you give a talk at your local school to children and

teachers about food allergy to help spread understanding of your condition or that of your child?

5.   Could you start up a local newsletter?

Writing and art therapy

Putting your thoughts, anxieties and fears down on paper is an excellent way of clearing your head, unburdening yourself, understanding your problems and charting your emotional progress. Consider finding an allergic pen friend, keeping a diary or even starting a 'blog', that is, an online web diary of your experiences of food allergy, which may well attract attention from other sufferers worldwide or find a good allergy discussion group on the internet, and regularly post messages.

Children can be encouraged to write stories or even make drawings, which you can then use to open up a discussion on their thoughts and feelings about their allergies.

Relaxation and breathing

Many people complain of being unable to relax, but there is more to unwinding than merely willing yourself to do so. Pampering by a hot bath, aromatherapy oils can help, as can a massage from a willing partner. Meditation, prayer and chanting are deeply relaxing; as are forms of yoga and healing martial arts such as t'ai chi. Find what works for you, and remember that relaxation takes practice.

For instant stress relief if you're feeling uptight or nervous, try a technique of 'expanding' your peripheral vision. Find a point opposite you, just above eye level, and keeping your eyes on that point, begin to slowly broaden your field of vision to notice more of what's on either side of the point, so that eventually you're paying attention to that which is visible in the corners of your eyes. You should begin to feel your breathing moving lower in your chest, slowing down, becoming deeper, and your facial muscles relaxing. This is very calming.

Indeed, learning to breathe correctly is of enormous value to relieve stress. Inhale deeply and slowly into the belly to the count of three, exhale evenly to the count of three, then pause for one and repeat. Yogic breathing while seated and focussing on a lit candle is very soothing.

If you suffer panic attacks, focussing on good breathing practice can reduce the symptoms caused by hyperventilation during acutely stressful moments.

Friends and family

The role of loved ones in your psychological care should never be underestimated.

Good friends...

You need around you positive people who can offer practical advice and emotional support, who can lift your gloom and bring laughter into your life when you feel there is none, and who make you feel understood. The most valuable are the people who know your needs, the implications of your illness, can act as your personal 'bodyguards' should your guard slip and who don't make any demands in return. The best friends to have are 'radiators', that is, reliable, there when you need them, able to provide you with warmth. They should be people you can turn to for help, especially when you are feeling overwhelmed or anxious about food allergy.

But that doesn't mean all your friends should be sweet and lovely all the time. You also need people who are unafraid to give you difficult truths when they apply to point out that you are foolishly taking risks with certain foods, or that you may benefit from seeking professional help with your mental health, for instance.

Shutting people out is a never win situation. Most who care for you will want to help in any way they can, so don't be too proud to ask for practical help or a shoulder to cry on. You may feel you want to protect family members from the burden of your illness, but, again, most prefer to be involved even if it's just by giving you a ride to the allergy clinic.

...and not so good friends

Understand that not everyone you meet, work with or are friendly with will be helpful or supportive, often due to ignorance not malice. Some people will not understand the reality of allergies, and will insist that 'allergies are all in the mind' because an article they once read said so, or they may think that you are being excessively fussy about your allergic child in restricting his or her diet. Upsetting as this may be, this will probably always be the way to some extent, and arguing the case may not always prove fruitful, or make you feel better. Some people will understand if you explain politely and clearly, but there will always be some who refuses to believe you or who will not listen.

All friends have their strengths and weaknesses, and a much valued confidant may not necessarily be the right one to turn to when you're suffering problems related to your allergy. There are three types to avoid when the going gets tough:

1. 'The Happy' – who trivialises your allergy and tells you not to be silly, that it's nothing to worry about.

2. 'The Hijacker' – who takes over and tells you about his problems with ill health when you ask for support with yours.

3. 'The Awfuliser' – who is alarmed at your condition and treats
    it like a crippling handicap or threatening death sentence.

Be aware of these, and of other people who make you feel
worse such as those who appear to enjoy the 'fuss' of your illness,
or who seem to be bored by or indifferent towards it.

Anonymous support

The internet revolution has seen a number of groups dedicated
to food allergy sufferers spring up online, see 'Useful Resources'
section.

People who live in secluded areas and feel isolated, those who
are disabled, or single parents of young children are among those
who find these groups of particular value but they can help anyone
who perhaps is shy or has difficulty with face-to-face contact, and
prefers the anonymity the world wide web and e-mail can offer.

Although groups can be extremely encouraging and supportive,
be sure to choose one with a knowledgeable moderator, who will
remove any controversial, offensive or dangerous postings. Stay
safe when posting messages online, and don't give away too much
personal information.

You may feel more comfortable talking to a stranger on the
telephone. Try a mental health helpline or other telephone support
organisation such as Aasra.

Professional help

Sometimes, stubborn psychological problems need to be referred
a step further.

Your doctor

Doctors are your first port of call if you're suffering symptoms of stress, depression, anxiety or are concerned with other areas of your or your child's psychological health. They are trained to see signs of emotional difficulties in their patients, and ideally placed to advise on possible private treatments or referrals.

Your dietitian

If you're anxious about food avoidance or nutrition, or wary or scared of foods a dietitian can help fill the gaps in your knowledge and offer excellent guidance and reassurance. Dietitians may also have a role to play in identifying and helping resolve possible eating disorders and aversions, as well as other food sensitivites such as intolerances.

Your allergy consultant

Your most complex queries can almost certainly be answered by your allergy consultant, with whom you should try to develop an active relationship. The more knowledge you demonstrate, and the more questions you ask of specialists, the more likely you will be given greater detail and reassurance. If you feel burdened by not knowing whether or not you are still allergic to a particular food, for instance, a consultant can arrange further testing.

'Talking' therapists

If your doctor feels you need more specialised help, referral for counselling or psychotherapy may be suggested.

There are few differences between the talking therapies, even though counselling sounds and is gentler and less demanding than psychotherapy. Both involve face-to-face meetings with a trained therapist to reach any number of end goals, depending entirely on the patient, such as the reduction of psychological distress and the promotion of emotional health.

Counsellors will listen to you, aim to identify with you and your dilemmas, help you clarify them in your mind, and perhaps give advice, although generally their aim is to guide you to discover your own answers to your problems through carefully guided discussion. Counsellors can, for instance, help patients cope and come to terms with difficult events like diagnosis.

Psychotherapists, of which there are many kinds, work similarly, but use more analytical approaches and explore difficulties in greater depth. They may work with those suffering from depression, anxiety and addictive behaviour disorders, those who are finding it difficult to adjust to allergic illness, those whose condition is impacting on many areas of their life, or anyone traumatised by an anaphylactic experience.

Make sure you have an assessment session, and discontinue any therapy with a specialist with whom you feel uncomfortable, being at ease with your counsellor is vital. Remember too that counselling is not easy, or a magic wand so expect positive changes but not miracles. Some people approach therapy expecting their stresses to be entirely removed, but therapists will not do this. They will arm you with coping mechanisms, not seek to abolish all your responses.

Professional therapy can work wonders with a whole family, when an allergic child is anxious and fearful of the threat of food. The key is to try to introduce and maintain a balance between a child's safety, and allowing the child to participate as much as possible in everyday activities typical of their age. A therapist can help you all towards this goal.

Cognitive Behaviour Therapy (CBT)

CBT is an objective psychotherapeutic approach which is less interested in what caused your emotional or psychological difficulties, and more concerned with how you handle your dilemmas. It challenges the negative thought patterns which may be causing your problems, helps you identify and understand them, equips you with coping skills, and implements changes to unhelpful thinking or behaviour. The therapy is structured, practical and result focused, unlike counselling which usually involves 'freer' conversation and a greater rapport with the therapist.

CBT might be right for those looking for help with a specific issue. It is useful for depression, phobias or stress, for example, where the emphasis may be on cognition or thinking; while for eating disorders or OCD, predominantly behavioural issues will be tackled.

Hypnotherapy

This is a psychotherapy which uses hypnosis; a state of deep relaxation and heightened awareness, which makes the mind more receptive to positive suggestion. It can help those suffering from low self esteem, phobias, panic, anxiety and OCD, to name a few.

Chapter 7

Nutrition and Health

You may be worried about the effects which reactions and dietary limitations have on your health. Rest assured that no matter how many food restrictions you have or how serious your symptoms, there is plenty you can do to keep yourself in optimal mental and physical shape.

Allergen-free nutrition

Living with food allergies generally means living on a restricted diet, and living on a restricted diet may compromise your nutrition. Usually, though, introducing wholesome replacement foods into your eating plans and making other modest changes will ensure you don't suffer any deficiencies.

It is important to remember that you should only exclude foods which you are certain cause a problem, preferably confirmed by testing and a diagnosis from an allergist, dietitian or doctor, and certainly not an alternative therapist or other non specialist.

This is especially important in young growing children, who can be very vulnerable to the effects of a restricted diet. Some parents become convinced that foods such as eggs, milk and citrus fruits aggravate their child's eczema, for example, and while this may be so in a few cases, it is essential you don't cut out these foods without specialist advice, or experiment with your child's diet in the absence of expert guidance. Food sensitivities are only sometimes to blame for aggravating asthma and eczema.

Tree nuts, peanuts and seeds

It's a bitter irony that these often dangerously allergic foods happen to be among the most nutritious available to us. Nuts and seeds are rich in proteins and essential fatty acids (EFAs), B vitamins, vitamin E, calcium and many important trace minerals.

Even if you are avoiding all varieties, however, there are unlikely to be any serious negative consequences on your health. Seafood, especially oily fish, offers a source of valuable EFAs, and you could look at including refined seed oils which should be free of allergenic proteins into your diet.

Other sources of trace minerals include barley, liver and seafood (for copper), brown rice, wholemeal bread, fish and chicken (for selenium), and meat, dairy, eggs, fish and soy (for zinc). Avocados are a good source of vitamin E, a natural anti-inflammatory and powerful antioxidant which may help mildly dampen allergy reactions.

Fish and seafood

This is rich in protein, minerals such as iodine and especially in the case of oily fish, omega-3 essential fatty acids, celebrated for their many beneficial effects, including cardiovascular functioning and psychological and mental wellbeing.

If you must omit seafood, incorporate olives, nuts and seeds such as flax, hemp, pumpkin and sunflower or their oils into your diet if you can. Liver and offal are also rich in omega 3s.

Dairy produce

Calcium intake is the main concern if you're allergic to dairy foods. Most soya milks are calcium enriched, but sardines and other bony fish, tofu, green vegetables (broccoli, spinach, lady's fingers/okra/bhindi), chickpeas and nuts are good alternative sources. Adequate vitamin D (from eggs, oily fish and sunlight's action on the skin) helps calcium's uptake by the body.

Yoghurt provides probiotic bacteria, which may help to maintain intestinal health. In its absence, you may like to consider other sources, like tempeh (fermented soy), fermented vegetables, like sauerkraut, and other fermented foods, like idli and dosa.

Prebiotics, that is, carbohydrates on which probiotics feed can encourage the growth and reproduction of health giving intestinal flora. Sources are bananas, members of the lily family (onion, garlic, asparagus), and some members of the daisy family (chicory, Jerusalem artichokes).

Wheat

Wheat is a good source of protein, starchy carbohydrates, fibre, B vitamins and minerals and therefore an excellent all round food. All its nutrients are vital to the body's many biological processes, but can be obtained from a varied diet of meat, dairy foods, eggs, nuts, pulses and seeds, fruit and vegetables and other cereals.

Try unrefined wholegrains such as brown rice, and experiment with nutritious grains such as amaranth, millet and quinoa, which rarely trigger allergies. Starchy vegetables such as potato, sweet potato and other tubers, and corn and polenta (Italian maize meal), constitute good carbohydrate replacements too.

Eggs

Eggs contain vitamins A and B, protein and some zinc, but having to eliminate them from your diet is unlikely to leave you deficient in a nutrient which cannot be obtained from an otherwise broad diet including meat, dairy or legumes.

Soy

A good vegetarian source of protein, and a useful source of calcium and other minerals. Although tough to avoid, especially if you eat a lot of ready meals and processed foods, omitting soy should not be problematic nutritionally. Other legumes such as peas and lentils can compensate.

Fruit and vegetables

These provide vitamins (especially vitamin C, a natural antihistamine), fibre (both soluble and insoluble) and some trace minerals. Dark or brightly coloured fruits and vegetables are also rich in antioxidant chemicals, helps in boosting immunity and protect against a wide range of illnesses, everything from colds to forms of cancer.

It's important to eat a selection of safe fruit and vegetables when you're excluding others, especially because research suggests that many allergy sufferers have reduced antioxidant status. One particular antioxidant of interest in allergy is quercetin, reputed to have a calming, anti-inflammatory effect; it is found in onions, apples and red grapes.

Most fruit allergy sufferers experience mild reactions to multiple fruits which are related to pollen sensitivity, and can eat tinned or cooked fruit, pasteurised juices and sometimes peeled fruits. Raw fruits rarely implicated in cross reactions with pollens and which are therefore usually safe include grapes, pomegranates, figs, many currants and berries. Citrus fruits are usually okay for adults, although some children can react to them.

Latex allergy sufferers with associated allergies to tropical fruits are more likely to find fruits which grow in cooler climates, such as apples, pears, berries, grapes and citrus fruits, more tolerable.

Those suffering reactions to fruits unrelated to either pollen or latex sensitivity are less likely to be sensitive to many fruits and so will have more choice in alternatives.

Nutritional deficiencies are unlikely if a wide range of vegetables (cooked if necessary) are also consumed.

Responses to vegetables are rare and generally resolved by cooking when pollen sensitivity is the cause, celery being an occasional exception. Having to avoid a particular type will not have nutritional consequences provided you eat many others.

However, those with tomato allergy may be missing out on the red antioxidant lycopene, which has anti cancer potential. Other, more moderate sources which you could include if you don't react to them are watermelon and guava.

Eating a healthy diet

So much is written nowadays about eating healthily that the consumer can easily become overwhelmed with the unnecessarily detailed and sometimes contradictory advice given. It's easy to form the impression that good nutrition is complex. It isn't. In reality, sticking to a few basic principles should ensure you maintain good dietary habits.

Possibly the most important is 'variety'. Try to eat as diverse a diet as possible within the parameters of your exclusions. Avoid coming to rely on any one 'safe' food which provides only a limited range of nutrients; over consumption can also increase your risk of becoming intolerant to a food.

How you eat is vital too. Take your time when you're selecting food, cooking it and most importantly eating it. Eat when you're calm and relaxed and can focus on your meal, not when you're rushed or anxious or distracted when mistakes and oversights are more likely. Remain quietly vigilant and on guard always. Take care not to become complacent about eating habits, continue to check ingredients and monitor your diet.

Also, don't skip meals, especially breakfast, you'll experience uncomfortable fluctuations in energy and blood sugar levels, and you'll be more vulnerable to casual snacking and grabbing possibly unsafe convenience foods on the go. Plan ahead, and always have healthy and safe foods with you should you be caught short and hungry.

And remember: just because you have a food allergy, doesn't mean you can't be passionate about food. Learn to cook new dishes. Interest yourself in food news and culinary innovations. Live life to enjoy taste experiences.

Essential foods

Several food groups are key to your diet.

Complex carbohydrates

These include all grains, and the foods based on them, such as pastas, breads and cereal products. Potatoes also fall into this category. Roughly eight to ten daily servings for adults and around four daily servings for children are recommended to ensure adequate intake of slow energy releasing carbohydrates and of fibre. A slice of bread, an egg sized potato, three tablespoons of cereal and two heaped tablespoons of rice count as a serving each.

Protein foods

Two to three servings of either meat, fish, eggs, beans, nuts or seeds are advised. A portion is equivalent to 100g of meat or fish, two eggs, three tablespoons of beans or a handful of nuts and seeds.

Fruit and vegetables

These should be taken as essential sources of carbohydrates, fibre, vitamins, minerals and antioxidant chemicals. Children should aim to consume five portions daily, and adults preferably more. A handful of berries, an apple, a banana, three tablespoons of peas or lentils, and two heaped tablespoons of salad are roughly equivalent to one portion.

Dairy foods

While not strictly essential, two or three servings of either milk, yoghurt or cheese are recommended by dietitians for both adults and children provided of course you don't have a dairy allergy (or a lactose intolerance – see Appendix 1). A matchbox sized chunk of cheese, a small pot of yoghurt or a small glass of milk each provide a serving.

Water / fluid

Two litres of water daily is the often quoted figure to which adults should supposedly all aspire, but the quantity depends on so many different factors like the size of the individual, the amount of activity undertaken, the temperature and environment, that it's misleading to put a firm figure on it. Less active children will not need so much water; very active adults will need a lot.

A good measurement of healthy and adequate hydration is the colour of the urine. Too dark signifies you may lack fluids, so aim to drink enough to keep your urine straw coloured. Water itself is the best hydrator, but fruit juices, squashes, sodas and milk all contain mostly water and count towards your quota. As do teas, coffees and colas, the dehydrating effects of the caffeine in these drinks is exaggerated by some complementary therapists but is very trivial in reality.

Alcoholic drinks, which dehydrate heavily, certainly do not count.

Non-essential foods

In moderation, other foods have their place in the context of a healthy diet, but take care not to overindulge.

Caffeine

Moderate caffeine consumption is safe for most, and perhaps even beneficial to people with asthma, but avoid drinking more than three to four cups of coffee daily in order to stay within recommended guidelines, and remember that black and green teas, cola, cocoa and chocolate products, as well as some painkillers, contain caffeine. Children should be protected from too much caffeine, and should not be allowed coffee until they are older.

Sugar

Cakes, biscuits, pastries, chocolate bars, sweets... most of us love occasional treats, and they're important for your psychological health, especially if you're feeling down about dietary limitations. Eat sugar sparingly, though no more than ten or even five per cent of your daily calories should come from sugar, which is roughly equivalent to 50g or twelve level teaspoons. Read labels carefully for added sugars.

Alcohol

Moderate alcohol consumption like a small glass of wine, or one or two glasses of beer is generally considered okay. Aside from the broad health risks of excessive alcohol consumption, as a food allergic person you need to take extra care as drinking can reduce your vigilance and numb your senses and responses, leaving you more liable to let your guard slip, thoughtlessly consume a reactive food, and also delay in recognising and treating symptoms of a reaction.

Convenience food and 'bad' fats

Although fat intake has no obvious direct relevance to food allergy sufferers, for other health reasons it's wise to limit your intake of junk foods and saturated fats, typically found in rich cuts of meat, dairy products such as butter and cream, and any number of desserts and sweet products.

Trans fats are a particular class of fats manufactured during hydrogenation which is a process which converts liquid vegetable oils into solid fats and margarines. Many researchers consider them unhealthier than saturated fats. Typically, trans fats are found in pastries, cakes, biscuits, convenience meat products, and take away foods.

Of course, some fats are needed in the diet, and unsaturated fats found in fish, nuts, seeds, avocados and vegetable oils such as olive oils are the best.

'Free-from' foods

As awareness of allergies and intolerances increases, there will be more 'free from' foods available. These will have their place, and will be very useful, but they may contain high levels of refined carbohydrates, fats and additives. Wheat-free products especially are worth examining carefully. Use modestly, and ask yourself whether the product is a good food in its own right. Would you eat it if you weren't suffering from food allergy?

Organic food

There is some evidence that organic food is healthier than non-organic, but the advantage may be very small. In those with oral allergies to fruit and vegetables, symptoms when eating organic versions may be milder because it's possible that pesticides used on non organic produce cause plants to manufacture greater quantities of 'defensive' allergens.

Supplementation

In certain circumstances, nutritional supplements may be suggested or advised but take your advice from your doctor or dietitian. Avoid supplementing without specialist advice, never assume you can compensate for omitted foods with vitamin pills, and don't use supplements as substitutes for skipped meals. Always verify supplements are allergen-free before taking them.

Do I need to see a dietitian?

Dietitians or professionally qualified nutritionists can advise on allergen avoidance, and on ensuring you follow a nutritionally adequate diet. Some have a special interest in food allergy.

A consultation could be useful if you have multiple allergies or additional dietary restrictions due to ethical or religious reasons, when following a healthy diet could be tricky. If, for example, you're a vegan with allergies to nuts, seeds and legumes, it's likely you'll need specialist advice on ensuring sufficient protein intake.

In most cases involving children, especially those with dairy allergy, seeing a dietitian or nutritionist for advice is very important.

Be very wary of unqualified therapists calling themselves nutritionists.

Health and your immune system

Given that in allergy your immune system is inappropriately

sensitive to certain proteins, looking after it may, some believe, reduce the severity of your responses and help you recover from reactions more quickly. Although the reasoning of this argument may be good, there's little evidence to suggest the effect is very strong in practice. Regardless, taking care of your overall health and immune system is certainly worthwhile for other reasons. Other than eating healthily, here are some additional tips:

1. Take regular exercise. Ensure it's something you enjoy, not find a chore. If the gym doesn't do it for you, find something which does. Just 30 minutes vigorous activity, three times a week, can help cardiovascular health.

2. Ditch the cigarettes and cigars, for too many reasons to mention, including their effect on the immune system.

3. Don't work excessively. We have a five-day, 35-hour week for a reason. Working through all your waking hours makes it impossible for you to savour much needed 'down-time'. Switch off your computer and your mobile, and go for a relaxing stroll or play with your children instead.

4. Keep stress levels low. Anxiety suppresses immunity. Yoga, meditation, massage, a soothing bath, sex, all help you to wind down, especially at the end of a working day.

5. Get your eight hours of shut-eye. Sleep deprivation can make you feel run down and lower your immune defences. Allergy sufferers need to keep as alert as possible. If you don't get a full night's sleep, take ten minute catnaps during the day.

6. Show emotion and express your feelings; bottling it all up is psychologically and physiologically damaging.

7. Breathe clean air. Minimise exposure to pollutants and chemical substances, both inside and outside the home. For instance, avoid jogging in rush hour or near main roads, and try using natural cleansers in the home, such as lemon juice.

8. And finally... laugh! Watch back-to-back episodes of favourite comedies or spend weekends with entertaining friends. Laughter is not the best medicine, but it is certainly a very good one and scientific research supports this.

Chapter 8
Treatments and Prevention

If only we could make all allergies go away when they materialised,
or, even better, stop them developing in the first place, then this
book might not be needed. Unfortunately, such medical progress
could be some time away.

Treatments

The science of treating food allergic individuals with a view to
reducing their future responses to triggers or curing them of their
allergic tendencies is still in its infancy. A handful of treatment
modalities exist, but none is entirely satisfactory.

Immunotherapy (IT)

The basic principle of immunotherapy also called desensitisation,
or specific immunotherapy (SIT) is to inject the sufferer with
weak but increasingly strong doses of dilute allergen in order to
'persuade' an over reacting immune system to accept and tolerate
exposure to the trigger. The doses are given weekly initially, and
for a few months, and then at spaces of a month or two for up to

four years. The conditions treated are presently limited principally to severe hay fever and dust mite allergy.

Some patients do well on IT, and pollen allergy sufferers often find their cross reactions to raw foods become milder.

On the negative side, the treatment is long, tedious, may not work, can trigger minor localised symptoms, and runs the risk of causing a more severe reaction.

Another form of IT, called sub-lingual immunotherapy (SLIT), uses diluted drops of allergen under the tongue, and is popular in parts of continental Europe. Some trials using SLIT for food allergy have been promising.

Immunotherapy is not widely available, and is normally only offered to those whose quality of life is severely compromised by their illness. This may change, though, and further research may eventually yield an effective partial treatment for food allergies, so that a small accidental exposure may not result in a reaction.

Enzyme potentiated desensitisation (EPD)

This is a somewhat controversial form of desensitisation which uses injections of dilute allergen in combination with an enzyme released by immune cells when they are stimulated.

It is used for a wide range of sensitivities, including chemical intolerances, food allergies, asthma and food intolerances. Although there have been a few positive reports of benefits with EPD, equally there have been cases of unpleasant side effects, and orthodox medicine does not acknowledge it as an affective allergy treatment. It is best avoided.

Sodium cromoglycate (Nalcrom)

This is a non steroidal anti inflammatory drug, which acts as a mast cell stabiliser, preventing the cells from releasing histamine in response to an allergen. However, it must be taken before exposure has taken place to have any effect.

It is mainly prescribed to asthma sufferers, who generally need to take the drug for some time in order to 'build up' its useful effects in the body. It can also be used on an 'as needed basis', for instance, before exercise in those suffering from exercise induced asthma.

Cromoglycate's use in food allergy is limited. It is used only exceptionally in patients who experience rapid reactions, largely because it does not always work. Its long term usefulness is also unclear, and so it cannot come close to substituting permanent food avoidance, unfortunately.

That said, it is sometimes prescribed to those who have delayed allergies, with symptoms such as eczema and urticaria in response to food, and infants or indeed adults who react to a wide range of foods are sometimes helped by it.

Anti-IgE drugs

The development of drugs to disable IgE antibodies in the blood is one of the most exciting areas of research into the prevention of food allergic reactions.

One, omalizumab (Xolair), has proved useful in allergic asthma and hay fever, but its potential for treating food allergies is less clear. Clinical trials have been subject to setbacks, and there are plenty of potential problems, such as the great expense, and the fact that it is less likely to be effective in those with multiple allergies.

Alternatives

Most so-called treatments available through alternative therapists are unproven and should be regarded with scepticism.

'Mind' therapies

Treatments like hypnotherapy and meditation may be of benefit to food allergic patients, but only in the reduction of the anxiety associated with the condition. Some have suggested that the severity of allergic responses can be reduced through such therapies, but objective studies are lacking to support this view.

Herbalism

Although some herbal remedies have been shown to have properties which can relieve asthma, eczema or hay fever, none is currently thought to have any use in food allergy, although this situation may change with further research. Some Chinese herbs or combinations of herbs may have potential, but it is too soon to be sure.

Homeopathy

This is based on the notion that 'like cures like', that a substance capable of producing a symptom can relieve that same symptom when administered heavily diluted or in minute doses. The highly respected British Society for Allergy and Clinical Immunology (BSACI) states that there is inadequate evidence for the effectiveness of homeopathic treatments in treating allergies, including food allergies.

Acupuncture

Although a possible treatment for pain relief and mood elevation, acupuncture's role in treating symptoms of food allergy has not been validated. Some studies indicating that it may mildly relieve wheezing and hay fever are modestly encouraging. In Chinese medical practice, it would normally be used in conjunction with herbal treatments. It is probably better avoided.

Nambudripad's Allergy Elimination Technique (NAET)

This is formulated on discredited diagnostic methods and Chinese principles of acupressure, and is increasingly popular in the US and France. It is based on a flawed perception of allergy being caused by blockages of 'energy flow', which ignores what is known about the immune system response. Dr Adrian Morris, a respected allergist from the UK, has dubbed NAET 'the most unsubstantiated allergy treatment proposed to date'. Avoid it.

Future treatments and cures

We do not have a cure for food allergy yet, but there are a number of exciting developments which could yield future treatments.

Anti-IgE drug development is still in its infancy, and new research may find some effective medicines in the next five or ten years.

Desensitisation research is ongoing, with studies aiming to desensitise children to common allergens such as dairy and nuts. A very small peanut desensitisation project in Cambridge, in the United Kingdom, successfully desensitised four children to peanut by giving them extremely tiny oral doses of peanut flour every day, which were increased very gradually over a period of six months, until several whole peanuts could be tolerated.

Another interesting avenue is FAST, or Food Allergy Specific Therapy. Classical immunotherapy (IT) cannot be used for food allergy, as the risk of anaphylaxis is too great. FAST uses 'deactivated' food allergens instead, which are safer. Research is ongoing.

Genetically modified (GM) food and crop science offer tantalising possibilities. So-called allergy free GM nuts have been produced, and selecting and nurturing strains of food which lack particular allergenic proteins is another path being explored in

Sweden, for instance, a country with a severe birch pollen apple syndrome problem, cultivating low allergen apple breeds has been investigated.

Perhaps less appealing but potentially more remarkable is research into the role parasitic worms play in allergy prevention, which is working on the idea that immune systems are kept too busy with internal parasites to 'bother' reacting to allergens. Deliberately infecting patients with these worms for therapeutic purposes is called helminthic therapy, and it is being researched for lots of immune diseases, such as celiac disease and asthma. If a chemical or biological trigger can be isolated and harnessed, a cure could be developed in the future... hopefully without needing to infect sufferers with wriggly guests.

Prevention

Our understanding of food allergy is not complete, and recommendations on how to prevent them in the unborn or the very young, or stop further ones developing in those already sensitised, should not be considered set in stone. Sadly, the research seems inconclusive in this area, and allergy experts are in occasional disagreement.

We know that inheritance is the most important factor in determining the likelihood of developing a predisposition towards allergy; if one parent is allergic, the likelihood is roughly one in three of a child being born with a tendency towards an allergy; if both are, the chance is two in three, approximately.

However, other factors also come into play such as diet, exposure to pets and dust mites, environmental conditions and overuse of antibiotics and so predicting the risks is subject to a wide margin of error, as allergy is an unpredictable science.

Prevention during pregnancy

If you, your partner or another of your children is food allergic, or there is a lot of allergic illness in your family, you will understandably be concerned about your unborn child.

The greatest worry is over peanut allergy. Expert guidelines on this issue vary, and are occasionally revised. Some experts suggest that women from atopic families may wish to avoid eating peanuts, in order to prevent any risk of their unborn baby being sensitised to allergenic proteins crossing the placental bloodstream which some researchers believe may occur in the second half of pregnancy, not only to nut proteins, but to those in milk and egg too.

While this is possible, others have suggested it may be just as likely that an unborn child might develop tolerance towards an allergen if exposed to it in the womb.

As it stands, there is no conclusive study, research or evidence to suggest that eating or not eating peanuts during pregnancy affects the chances of your unborn child developing a peanut allergy. Many nations' health agencies are now advising women not to worry unduly about this issue, so the advice is to consume peanuts as a part of a healthy diet if you wish to do so, unless otherwise instructed by your allergy specialist, or of course unless you are allergic to them yourself.

If you are concerned about allergies to other foods, seek the advice of your allergist and perhaps a dietitian. Avoidance of milk in pregnancy, for instance, could compromise calcium intake, and should not be undertaken without professional supervision. However, again, there is no firm evidence to suggest that avoidance of other allergens is beneficial in pregnant women, and there is some to suggest that restricted diets in pregnancy are associated with lower birth weights and impaired weight gain in babies.

Eating a full and wide ranging healthy diet when expecting a baby appears the best advice at present.

Avoiding active and passive smoking during pregnancy does lessen the risk to your unborn child, however, and you should consume a varied and balanced diet, with adequate amounts of iron and folic acid, especially. Avoid alcohol, exposure to pollution and strong chemicals, and excessive contact with pets or house dust.

Take particular care to avoid any of your own food allergens, if you have any. The more reactions you have during pregnancy the more likely your child may inherit a disposition towards a similar allergy.

Prevention during breastfeeding and the early months

Once your child is born, if you can, breastfeed exclusively for at least four months, but preferably six, and try to continue non exclusively beyond, as all this helps prevent the development of food allergies (and eczema) in children with a family history of allergic illness.

With regard to your own diet, again some experts may advise that you avoid certain foods such as peanuts while breastfeeding. However, latest research shows there is no evidence to suggest that eating or not eating peanuts when breastfeeding affects your baby's chances of developing a peanut allergy. Unless you are allergic to peanuts or are specifically advised to avoid them by your allergist, you may consume them as part of a healthy diet. The same goes for other allergenic foods. It is not recommended to restrict a breastfeeding mother's diet without very good reason.

If breastfeeding is not possible or desired, an extensively hydrolysed, or hydrolysate, formula feed may be recommended by your doctor or paediatric specialist if your baby is at high risk of developing food allergies. These are made from cow's milk, but because the proteins are mostly broken down into non-allergenic fragments, they are thought to reduce the risk of sensitisation. (They are not suitable for already sensitised babies, however, as some whole proteins may survive the hydrolyzing process.)

Amino acid or elemental/hypoallergenic formulas are not made from cow's milk, and are considered safe and effective for severely atopic babies (or those with an extremely strong cow's milk allergy).

The introduction of a non-hydrolysed cow's milk formula before six months, and especially before four months, should be avoided, as this is known to increase the risk of your baby developing a milk protein allergy. There is also no place for soy or goat's milk formula in the primary prevention of allergy, as a susceptible baby is as likely to become allergic to these as to cow's milk.

Whether breastfed or not, again, protect your new baby from smoke and other allergens, but don't be paranoid about maintaining a scrupulously sterile environment in the home, too much extreme cleanliness may have the opposite effect to that desired. Be clean, but not obsessively so.

Is my baby developing a food allergy?

The most common food allergy in new babies is cow's milk, usually because they have been sensitised to a cow's milk formula given to them when breastfeeding has been delayed after birth. Some symptoms to look out for include:

1. Eczema.
2. Urticaria, itching and rashes.
3. Reflux, regurgitation and vomiting.
4. Diarrhoea or constipation or abnormal stools.
5. Wheezing and respiratory distress.

Depending on the severity, either call emergency services or take your baby to the doctor should he have any of these symptoms. If milk allergy is diagnosed, extensively hydrolysed formula milks will probably be recommended, but if the allergy is extremely severe or if formula milk is not working, an elemental formula, which is totally free of any cow's protein, may be advised.

Soy formula should not be given except under very particular and rare circumstances.

Breast milk remains the best choice for the cow's milk allergic baby, but because cow's milk proteins can be detected in the mother's milk, in serious cases the mother may need to restrict her own consumption of cow's milk protein. This has been shown to help cases of infant eczema and digestive illness due to cow's milk protein. In this case, the advice of a dietitian must be sought to advise on the maternal diet.

Prevention during weaning

Weaning should be delayed until at the very least four months, but preferably six months, as the World Health Organization recommends.

The introduction of solid foods should be done gradually and individually at six months. A new food can be introduced every several days, so that any reactions to it can be more easily identified.

The issue of when exactly to introduce particular foods into the diets of infants has been the subject of much debate.

For a while it has generally been considered better to begin with cooked foods unlikely to trigger allergies such as pears, pureed root vegetables (carrot, sweet potatoes), green vegetables and, later, meats. The advice has been to start with small amounts of one food, and gradually increase, before introducing another food after several days.

Once these have been incorporated, from around seven months, other foods can begun to be given, such as grains (oats, wheat), pulses (peas, daals, beans) and dairy foods.

Previously, it was thought a wise precaution that the introduction of highly allergenic foods (such as egg, nuts and fish) should be delayed, but it appears there is no evidence either way as to whether this helps prevent the development of food allergies or not.

And so, unless otherwise advised by your allergist, who may have up-to-date advice and information, at present there are no specific recommendations to delay the introduction of any particular allergenic food beyond six months.

If, after speaking to your healthcare provider, you decide to wean before six months, avoid giving your baby any highly allergenic foods at first, and until he or she reaches six months. Wean them on foods unlikely to trigger allergies.

With all prepared foods, remember to read labels, and aim to give your child as pure a diet as possible, free from artificial colourings and preservatives.

Also, always avoid introducing new foods when a child is unwell.

If your infant already has a food allergy or eczema, he has a higher risk of developing peanut allergy, so in this case it is worth speaking to your allergy specialist before introducing peanuts into his diet.

Remember to never give whole nuts to infants, as they are a choking hazard.

Is my infant developing a food allergy?

Closely monitor your infant throughout weaning and beyond for allergic symptoms. Consider keeping a food/symptom diary, which may be useful in identifying potential triggers to ill health and discomfort. Keep a daily record of everything you feed your child; especially make note of when new foods are introduced, and any symptoms. Signs to watch out for include:

1. Urticaria, skin blotches, eczema.
2. Swelling anywhere on the body.
3. Colic, vomiting, diarrhoea, constipation, abnormal stools.
4. Persistent rhinitis or nasal symptoms.
5. Regular wheezing or coughing.
6. Ear infections, discharge or discomfort.
7. Refusing to breastfeed, food rejection or obvious problems in eating.
8. Any other unusual symptoms or unexplained changes in behaviour.

If symptoms present themselves, see your doctor promptly.

Prevention in later childhood and adulthood

There is little research on preventing new or additional food allergies developing beyond infancy, and again it is difficult to give firm advice.

Maintaining a good, varied diet can only benefit your health, so ensure that diet of yours and that of your child is nutritious.

Avoiding tobacco, alcohol and unnecessary drugs and medicines is also likely to help; as is reducing your exposure to other allergens.

If you work in food processing, ensure you are protected with overalls, gloves and face masks where practical.

Gut integrity

Many of the ideas in allergy prevention centre on maintaining a healthy digestive system.

An adequate intake of probiotics and prebiotics (see pg. 107) may help people of all ages, according to several Scandinavian studies, although the possible mechanisms are not yet understood.

Some studies have suggested that a diet rich in omega 3 essential fatty acids (found in oily fish, linseed, walnuts, pumpkin seeds and sunflower seeds) can help reduce the production of allergy antibodies, and it is known that essential fatty acids help the gut membranes.

Abnormally high gut permeability, dubbed leaky gut syndrome (LGS), is another possible cause of greater susceptibility to food allergies, although some experts are unconvinced by this idea, which tends to be popular among alternative therapists. In LGS, the gut wall, which usually allows only small digested food molecules to pass through it into the bloodstream, supposedly becomes inflamed or irritated, allowing larger, undigested protein molecules to enter, possibly sensitising the individual or triggering an immune response. Some have suggested that by preventing LGS, atopic individuals may reduce their risks of developing further allergies.

Factors which may contribute to LGS, and which therefore may be worth avoiding where possible, include:

1. Medicines, painkillers and drugs.
2. Alcohol, tobacco and excessive caffeine.
3. Refined sugar, processed foods, food additives.
4. Very spicy foods (chilli, hot curry).
5. Enzymic fruits (papaya/pawpaw, mango, pineapple) on an empty stomach.
6. Chronic stress.
7. Environmental toxins.
8. Food poisoning.

It is worth getting any sporadic or chronic digestive troubles you suffer from such as irritable bowel syndrome (IBS), indigestion, or heartburn, investigated and resolved, as their underlying causes may in some cases make you also more susceptible to allergies and food intolerances. One interesting study from Austria found that antacid or indigestion pills, made food allergic reactions more likely, possibly because they interfere with the breakdown and neutralisation of potentially allergenic proteins in the digestive system. As so often is the case in medicine, it may be better to investigate and cure the root cause, rather than merely treat or mask any symptoms you're experiencing.

Maintaining good eating habits is highly recommended; don't skip meals, don't eat on the go, do eat slowly and deliberately, don't overeat in one sitting, don't drink too much alcohol or acidic fluids (wine, orange juice) with your meals, and always avoid extreme or fad weight loss diets.

Non Allergic Food Intolerances

Not all adverse reactions to food are true food allergies. While the subject of this book is food allergy in the strictest sense, it is worth covering some other types of reactions briefly, as many readers or their children may have other responses to food which are not strictly allergic, but may be a cause for health concern nevertheless. These are covered more fully in the book, *Living with Food Intolerance*, by this book's author.

What is a food intolerance?

A food intolerance is a delayed adverse reaction to food, which can sometimes occur as soon as an hour after consumption of the problem food, but more commonly occurs several hours or even days afterwards. Unlike a food allergy, it is not rapid or sharp or alarming, but it is slow to progress and never directly life threatening. Usually in food intolerance, the immune system is not involved. Typical symptoms might be stomach upsets, digestive disturbance, diarrhoea, bloating, lethargy, tiredness, headaches, chronic skin problems and any number of other general complaints.

As these symptoms can often have a number of causes, identifying a food intolerance is not always easy.

It is worth reiterating that you should never casually remove foods from your diet which you suspect may be causing a reaction. It is vital you consult your doctor or a dietitian if you suspect a problem. Don't experiment with food exclusion on a whim.

Diagnosis in some cases can be very difficult, and for unusual reactions it is best attempted by means of a carefully controlled and monitored exclusion diet – see Appendix 2.

Lactose intolerance

This is the inability or reduced ability to digest lactose, the sugar found in milk and milk products such as yoghurt and cheese and is the most common food intolerance in the world.

It is caused by a lack of the enzyme lactase in the body, which breaks down lactose. Without lactase, lactose passes through the system undigested, providing food for bacteria in the gut. This process creates gas and draws water into the gut leading to symptoms of bloating, wind, diarrhoea and abdominal pain, from a few minutes to two hours after consumption.

There are two forms:

1. Primary lactose intolerance, which is inherited and permanent, and typically begins between the ages of five and 20, due to natural reduction in lactase production. The reduction can be partial, meaning a small amount of dairy food can be tolerated, or it can be more complete, meaning little or no dairy food can be tolerated.

2. Secondary lactose intolerance, which occurs when you have gastroenteritis, food poisoning or other illnesses of the gut, and can affect people of all ages. It usually resolves after a

period of abstinence from lactose and when the underlying illness has cleared up.

Around 70% of the world's population is lactose intolerant. Asian and African groups are particularly affected, with 20-70% of Indians (depending on ethnic group and geographical area), around 80% of central Asians, and 98% of Thais with some degree of lactose intolerance.

Many people instinctively self diagnose their lactose intolerance, but your doctor can conduct breath or stool tests to confirm it.

It is not a 'disease' as such, and while it is unpleasant to experience symptoms, it is generally harmless. Any 'treatment' is normally just a matter of reducing consumption of lactose containing foods by trial and error until no side effects are experienced.

All the foods listed on pg 51 are the ones to be wary of, but some dairy foods are naturally lower in lactose than others. For instance, live yoghurt and very hard or fatty cheeses are usually low in it; low fat or white/soft cheeses may have a little more; fresh milk has a lot. Low lactose milk and cheeses imported from Australia are now on the market. For babies, there are low lactose formula milks available.

There are also some enzyme supplements which may be taken with a dairy containing meal to help digestion but it is important you speak to your doctor about these first as they may not be suitable for everyone.

If you are drastically altering your diet due to lactose intolerance, see a nutritionist or dietitian for advice.

Celiac disease

This is a lifelong disease caused by a particular intolerance to gluten, which is the protein found in wheat and some other grains.

In sufferers, gluten causes an auto immune or 'self attacking' response in the intestine, which damages the gut, preventing it from absorbing nutrients properly. Symptoms of undiagnosed celiac disease vary, but include ongoing diarrhoea, bloating, constipation, tiredness, malnutrition, weight loss, mouth ulcers, anaemia, lactose intolerance and infertility. Many sufferers feel almost constantly unwell, and in children there are usually signs of failure to grow fully or 'thrive'.

Up to 1% of Western populations have celiac disease, but it is heavily under diagnosed and often misdiagnosed as irritable bowel syndrome (IBS). It is rarer in Asian and African nations, because wheat is not such a staple part of the diet, but may affect around 1 in 300 Indians, mostly in the northern parts of the country, where wheat is more common. However, with an increased tendency to consume Western foods, it is likely to become more prevalent.

There are very good tests for celiac disease like blood tests followed by an internal biopsy. These are extremely reliable and the only possible way to diagnose the condition. Speak to your doctor if you would like to be tested, and he may refer you to a gastroenterologist.

Treatment is through a very strict gluten exclusion diet, meaning no wheat, rye or barley, or products containing them. The Celiac Society for Delhi has more information, including sources of gluten-free produce.

Irritable Bowel Syndrome (IBS)

IBS is a common, functional gut disorder, with symptoms of diarrhoea or constipation or both, abdominal pain, bloating, flatulence and bathroom urgency.

Stress, overwork, and a poor diet may all be involved in IBS. It is not usually caused by a food intolerance, but it is the case that people with IBS have bowels which are over-sensitive to food in general. Foods which upset many people, such as fatty foods, very spicy foods, strong coffee, or gas generating foods such as daals, cereals and fruits, can cause more problems if you have IBS.

You may need to adjust your intake of insoluble fibre. This is found in wholemeal flours and breads, whole grains, brown rice and bran cereals. If you consume a lot, it may be worth trying to reduce your intake, and replacing it with soluble fibre, which is found in oats, daals, fruits and green vegetables.

It's a good idea to keep a daily diary of symptoms, diet and life events if you have IBS, which can help you identify what brings on symptoms.

Take the time to eat healthy and regular meals, and to relax and enjoy your food, without over indulging. Lead a balanced life, with plenty of exercise and rest.

If you or your nutritionist suspect certain food intolerances, it may be worth attempting an exclusion diet, though this should never be done without expert supervision, support and advice. Wheat intolerance is a common trigger for IBS symptoms in the West.

Fructose malabsorption / intolerance

Fructose is a type of sugar found in either free or bound form in table sugar, honey, fruit, fruit juices, some dried fruits, some vegetables and wheat.

Some people cannot process large quantities of fructose in the gut, and experience symptoms very similar to those in lactose intolerance when they consume a lot of fructose at a time. This is especially true of people with IBS, and may explain why fruits and wheat are often reported to be a problem in this condition.

Alcohol intolerance

This is common among many Asian peoples due to a deficiency of a detoxification enzyme which breaks alcohol down, causing symptoms of facial flushing, nausea and other symptoms normally associated with heavier drinking. Those with chronic allergic conditions such as asthma, rhinitis and urticaria may find their symptoms worsen after alcohol consumption, and they should limit their intake. Alcohol can also cause headaches in susceptible people.

Caffeine sensitivity

This stimulant, found in coffee, tea, cola drinks, chocolate and some painkillers, can have some benefits. It is a mild painkiller, it can help asthma symptoms, and it can revive energies. But it can also bring on unpleasant symptoms in certain people in very modest amounts. These include nausea, anxiety, headache, sweating, migraines, irregular heartbeat and sleep disruption. Many low caffeine or caffeine-free options exist, and it is worth experimenting with them if you think you are caffeine sensitive.

Biogenic amine sensitivity

The biogenic (or vasoactive) amines are a class of very active chemicals which can affect all people, sometimes with symptoms which are not unlike real food allergy reactions, such as urticaria, wheezing, nausea, flushing and others, and also sharp headache, the symptom which perhaps they are most known for.

Histamine is a biogenic amine, and reactions involving naturally occurring histamine in food are often confused with allergic reactions. Foods rich in histamine include strong European cheeses (Parmesan, Roquefort), red wines and certain highly flavoured fish (tuna, mackerel, especially when it has been improperly stored). Some vegetables too, such as spinach and eggplant, are high in histamine.

Other biogenic amines, such as tyramine and phenylethylamine, are found in many of the foods in which histamine is also found, but also in fermented foods such as soy-based foods, pickled foods, chocolate and mature cheeses. These may also cause headaches in some people.

Monosodium Glutamate (MSG) sensitivity

This is a flavour enhancer widely used in Chinese food and also naturally occurring in very flavourful foods such as strong cheeses, savoury snacks, sauces (especially soy sauce), stocks and stock cubes. It has been blamed for a number of allergy like intolerance reactions, such as nausea, increased pulse, flushing, headache, dizziness, urticaria and so on, but studies have not been able to find fully convincing evidence for this. It is possible that some people with asthma may react to MSG, but even this is still uncertain.

Sulphite sensitivity

About 1-2% of asthmatics react to sulphite preservatives in foods such as cold meats and fish, alcoholic beverages such as white wine, dried food such as fruit and fish, prepared salads, and baked goods, sometimes severely enough to trigger anaphylaxis. The cause is thought to be sulphur dioxide which is released from the sulphites when they're consumed, although the mechanism is not understood. Other possible reactions include headaches, urticaria, and angioedema. In people with IBS, sulphites may worsen digestive upsets.

Reactions to food colourings

Artificial food colourings make food more visually appealing, but there are a number of health concerns with some of them, some of which are disputed. As far as food sensitivities go, there are several possible reactions to many of the colourings, and those with allergies may be more susceptible to them.

The symptoms and reactions which have been associated with colourings are wide ranging, and include shortness of breath, wheezing, urticaria, angioedema, eczema, migraine, digestive upsets, visual disturbances and many other idiosyncratic reactions.

If you have asthma or are sensitive to aspirin, you may be more vulnerable to the effects of some of the colours, so they are worth avoiding in these cases.

However, overall, it is thought that a very small percentage of children and an even smaller percentage of adults will react to them.

Here are some of the main colourings which have been implicated in causing reactions, together with their European (E number) name, alternative names and US name, where applicable or available.

1. Tartrazine (E102 / Food Yellow 4 / Acid Yellow 23 / FD&C Yellow 5).
2. Quinoline Yellow (E104 / Food Yellow 13).
3. Yellow 2G (E107 / Food Yellow 5 / Acid Yellow 17).
4. Sunset Yellow (E110 / Food Yellow 3 / FD&C Yellow 6).
5. Carmoisine (E122 / Food Red 3).
6. Amaranth (E123 / Food Red 9 / FD&C Red 2).
7. Ponceau 4R (E124 / Food Red 7).
8. Erythrosine (E127 / Food Red 14 / FD&C Red 3).
9. Red 2G (E128 / Food Red 10).
10. Allura Red (E129 / Food Red 17 / FD&C Red 40).
11. Patent Blue V (E131/ Food Blue 5).

12. Indigo Carmine / Indigotine (E132 / Food Blue 1 / FD&C Blue 2).
13. Brilliant Blue (E133 / Food Blue 2 / FD&C Blue 1).
14. Brilliant Green BS / Green S (E142 / Food Green 4 / FD&C Green 4).
14. Black PN (E151 / Food Black 1).
15. Brown FK (E154 / Food Brown 1).
16. Brown HT (E155 / Food Brown 3).

There has been shown to be a link to hyperactivity in some children with Tartrazine, Quinoline Yellow, Sunset Yellow, Caromoisine, Ponceau 4R and Allura Red, when consumed with the preservative sodium benzoate. This may be the case with other colourings too.

Note that the wording 'no artificial colours' on a product does not necessarily exclude all colours, as cochineal and annatto, for example, are both derived naturally, cochineal from a particular type of female scale insect, and annatto from the pulp surrounding the seed of the achiote plant. There have been one or two reports of reactions to these.

Other colours which are considered safe, and even beneficial, are curcumin (derived from turmeric), riboflavin (vitamin B2), chlorophyll (which imparts green colour to plants), copper chlorophyll, caramel, carotene, lutein, canthaxanthin, beetroot red, anthocyanin, paprika and saffron.

Reactions to benzoic acid / benzoates

These are preservatives found in some beverages, baked goods, frozen foods, confectionery, cheeses, marinated fish, fruit products and assorted processed foods. They have occasionally been implicated in hyperactivity (as with sodium benzoate – see food colourings above), as well as symptoms of wheezing, urticaria, angioedema and other allergy like reactions. Children sensitive to food colourings and adults sensitive to aspirin may have more trouble with the benzoates.

Food induced rhinitis/conjunctivitis

This is a runny nose/weeping eyes triggered by certain strong foods such as horseradish, raw garlic, spices, chillies, for instance. This is quite normal.

Food toxicity

Wild fish and shellfish can absorb toxic algae, resulting in unpleasant gastrointestinal and feverish symptoms should you then eat the contaminated food, something often mistaken for fish allergy.

Psychological food aversions

These are responses caused by the mind. Some people can mistakenly convince themselves that a certain food triggers unpleasant symptoms when in fact the problem is psychological, and they have developed an emotional aversion to a food, with very real physical symptoms. This can be very hard to diagnose, and requires a specialist dietitian.

Medical Tests and Diagnoses

If you or your child have been experiencing symptoms of food allergy, a full professional health evaluation must be carried out. Your doctor may make a referral to an allergy consultant or clinic for professional assessment. However, some doctors have only a modest understanding of food allergy, and may believe the problem is not to do with food, or may suggest a number of foods are eliminated from the diet. If you are not satisfied, do explain to your doctor that you feel it is serious, and don't be afraid of seeking a second opinion if you feel you need to.

Food allergy diagnosis

Diagnosis of food allergy can only be made with any degree of confidence by a trained clinical doctor or allergist using a process which combines a complete assessment of you or your child, with a consideration of the symptoms, a medical and family history, and good but by no means perfect laboratory and out-patient testing procedures. In some cases, you or your child may be asked to submit to a food 'challenge'.

Other past or present allergic conditions, such as asthma or pollen sensitivity, must be considered, as must seasonal or environmental sensitivities or reactions, possible occupational exposure to food products, and other reactions to foods, such as intolerances. Physical tests of lung functioning, and examinations of the eyes, nose and skin, can help your specialist determine which, if any, tests should be undertaken.

Questions you may be asked

Before a consultation, it is a good idea to prepare for the questions you may be asked by a specialist or doctor. Write it all down if it helps. Here are some things medics may ask you:

1. How often do you or your child experience symptoms?
2. How quickly do they start after you or your child eat the problem food?
3. What are the symptoms, how severe are they, and how long do they last?
4. Have you taken / given any medication for the symptoms and has it worked?
5. Does anyone else in your family experience symptoms?
6. Does anyone else in your family have allergies?

Skin prick testing (SPT)

SPT involves placing a drop of diluted allergen onto the skin of the forearm, then piercing the skin through the drop with a tiny needle. Itching within minutes, and the development of a swollen red wheal at the site, are indicative of a positive reaction; the larger the wheal, the stronger the response. Because such a tiny amount of allergen is used, SPT is extremely safe.

A positive response to a food allergen only sometimes means

you are allergic to it. You may have a positive SPT to an allergen which causes no reaction in the context of everyday exposure, or even to an allergen to which you reacted as a child, but have since outgrown.

A negative response is more valuable diagnostically, as it usually signifies you are not allergic. False negatives can occur, however, if your reaction is weak or delayed, you are taking antihistamines, or in the case of fruit or vegetables, some of whose allergens are unstable.

The accuracy of a positive SPT is around 55%; with a negative, it is 95%+. Some allergens, such as soy or apple, produce less reliable results; others, like fish and nuts, are more trustworthy.

SPT is suitable for all ages, and can be a useful contributor towards a confident diagnosis.

Blood testing

Various tests may be used to ascertain IgE levels to individual allergens present in your blood, including some called RAST and CAP.

Negative results are fairly reliable (around 90%), though false negatives are possible, especially if you have already excluded the suspect from your diet. Positive blood tests have a reliability of just above 50%, and can only contribute towards or help confirm a diagnosis, but never provide one exclusively of other tests or factors. Equally, they cannot generally give a reliable indication of the severity of any possible allergy.

Home blood testing

Some home testing kits for IgE antibodies are becoming available from private laboratories, pharmacists or on the world wide web online. A few provide immediate positive or negative results to a specific allergen; others require you to return a drop of blood for analysis.

While many of these are clinically correct in principle, a diagnosis reached on the basis of such a test in the absence of a professional consultation is not advised. Blood analyses can only ever form one piece of the allergy puzzle, therefore home testing cannot be recommended, at least not in isolation.

Exclusion diet

Often called an elimination diet, this is a diagnostic diet which aims to remove the suspect foods from your diet for a period of, say, a fortnight, or until symptoms disappear, and then reintroduce foods individually to see whether they return and which foods cause them to return.

It is rarely used in allergy diagnosis, and only when slow and delayed and non-life threatening symptoms, such as eczema, are experienced. It cannot be used to test for acute and severe reactions. It is more common in the diagnosis of some food intolerances, when it may be used by both dietitians and allergists.

It is vital you never attempt an exclusion diet on your own, as they are extremely difficult to plan, monitor and interpret. They are also sometimes very tough to stick to, so require a lot of motivation.

Challenge testing

A food allergy can be indicated if symptoms appear when you are challenged with the food, that is, you are asked to consume it especially after you have previously eliminated it from your diet.

1. Open challenging means you're aware of what you're being challenged with, and it is not reliable.

2. Single blind challenging means the tester is aware of what

you're being challenged with and you are not, which is better, but still not perfect.

3. Double blind challenging which is considered the 'gold standard' means neither of you are aware, removing all possible bias.

Challenge testing is time consuming, expensive, often risky, and it can be difficult to effectively disguise the appearance, taste and texture of foods in blind testing. As there is no universally accepted protocol on precisely how challenges ought to be administered, various techniques and systems are used.

A once popular procedure was to offer food disguised within a gelatine capsule, though this has fallen out of favour as it bypasses the oral membranes. Occasionally, the food may be 'hidden' within another food, such as a soup or a biscuit. However, this 'masking' may not provide an accurate reflection of how a food may normally be consumed, and so some testers have concluded that it's better to give the food in a form in which the patient would expect to encounter it in practice.

Typically, exposure is gradual at first, with perhaps a small dose being applied to your skin or lip, and then into the mouth, and then by ingestion of increasing amounts. Each stage is separated by at least ten minutes, while any possible reactions are carefully monitored.

If the challenge is positive at any stage, a positive diagnosis can be confidently made.

In the event of a negative challenge, a larger portion of the food may be openly given to confirm the diagnosis and offer reassurance to the patient. A good clinic will often 'chase' a negative diagnosis, to ensure that the patient has reincorporated the once suspect food back into their diet, and is not suffering any adverse effects.

Food challenges cannot usually be performed on those who have asthma or who may be at risk of anaphylaxis. They are only undertaken under close scrutiny, with resuscitation equipment and medication at hand.

Forms of challenge testing can also be useful when a patient suspects that an allergy may have been outgrown, wishes to reintroduce a doubtful food, or would like to check the safety of a potential cross reactor, or even the cooked or raw versions of the food, when a reaction to only one is confirmed.

OAS

Diagnosis of hay fever is typically made through circumstantial and symptomatic evidence. If you experience severe rhinitis and conjunctivitis during the pollen seasons, for example, a doctor may confidently suspect you have hay fever to the relevant pollen. Where there is doubt, SPTs for specific pollens may be performed, and these can help indicate potential cross reacting foods.

The fruit and vegetable allergens associated with OAS may also be tested for, but because they are prone to breaking down, fresh rather than stored sample extracts produce more reliable results, and many allergists are increasingly using them, adopting a modified SPT technique called Prick plus Prick testing (or Scratch plus Scratch). Here, the test food is first pricked, and then the patient's forearm is pricked, thereby introducing into the skin a fresh extract gathered on the tip of the lancet.

Latex allergy and food cross reactions

Latex allergy can be diagnosed effectively through blood testing, but similar testing for associated food allergies appears to be poor at indicating triggers. In one study, only a third of latex allergics reporting symptoms to cross reacting fruits tested blood positive to those fruits.

Alternative tests

There are a number of unreliable, unproven or questionable tests offered by alternative therapists, unqualified professionals and private laboratories which sometimes appeal to people who are desperate for a diagnosis.

Practitioners can be extremely persuasive. You may be told that orthodox diagnostic tests are not 100% accurate, something the medical profession freely admits. You may also be told that the doctors are dismissive of food allergy and unsympathetic towards its sufferers which is an unfair and sweeping generalisation.

Another complicating factor is that some therapists adopt vague or inaccurate definitions of both food allergy and food intolerance, and don't always draw an agreed distinction between the two, leaving the patient confused as to what, exactly, is being tested for.

Some of the tests available include:

1. Applied kinesiology – This is where samples of the tested food are placed under the tongue or in the hand, and the arm muscles are tested for strength, a weakened response being supposedly indicative of sensitivity. There is no scientific evidence that kinesiology works.

2. Electrodermal skin testing techniques and systems including Vega, BEST, Dermatron, Listen and Quantum. These look for changes in skin resistance in response to allergens held within an electrical circuit. The results are unreliable and variable, and there is no proof the systems work.

3. Hair or fingernail analyses – These look for assorted mineral traces, from which conclusions about food sensitivities are drawn. Again, there is nothing to support their use in the realm of food sensitivities.

4. Cytotoxicity testing – An unproven technique of adding allergens to the patient's blood cells in a test tube, and monitoring responses to reach deductions about sensitivity.

5. IgG testing – This is a blood test which looks for levels of a type of antibody called IgG, which is 'gentler' than the IgE involved in true food allergy. It is used to test for delayed allergies and food intolerances. Despite some initial interest in IgG testing, there seems to be very little evidence that the test offers any useful information, as people can have high levels of IgG and show no symptoms of ill health. It can be extremely expensive and most experts working in allergy and intolerance consider the test to have no use in diagnosing a food sensitivity at all.

6. Pulse testing – This is based on the idea that your rate of heartbeat rises after you eat a food to which you are allergic or intolerant. There is no evidence whatsoever for this.

The results from these tests follow a strikingly similar pattern. One or both of wheat or dairy foods are commonly identified as culprits, and to these will be added other supposed allergens, often including obscure foods, in order to give the impression of precision to the patient. In fact, multiple and unrelated food allergies are fairly rare, and the restricted diets demanded by the results of such tests can put you or your child at risk of malnutrition. Equally, a false negative result to a particular food can result in unsafe reassurance that you are not allergic to a possible trigger.

None of these tests is reliable, then. All are either clinically unproven or have been discredited by independent medical studies, facts which the practitioner is unlikely to tell you.

Ask your doctor for a reputable private clinic or hospital which can undertake skin prick, blood or challenge testing, and be wary of anything else.

Appendix 3
Food Families

Cross reactions often occur between related foods. The following can give an indication of those you might need to avoid should you be allergic to one or more family members.

Plant foods

Any not categorised below are likely to form one member groups, with no common close edible relatives. The examples include amaranth, capers, coffee, drumstick (moringa), elderberry, linseed, ginkgo biloba, ginseng, grapes, kiwi, lychee, olives, papaya, peppercorns, persimmon, pineapple, poppy seed, sesame, sweet potato, tea and vanilla, as well as many of the tree nuts. However, being an 'only child' is not predictive of a food's reactive potential. Kiwis are highly allergenic, for instance, while tea is not.

Besides, cross reactions are also possible between unrelated foods. The tree nuts are a good example. Although many are individualists, they often cross react with one another, and with peanut, a legume, and almond, a rose member. It's a similar picture with many seeds.

Banana family: Banana, plantain.

Carrot Family: Ajwain/carom, angelica, aniseed, asafoetida/ hing, caraway, carrot, celeriac, celery, chervil, coriander, cumin, dill, fennel, Indian penny wort, lovage, parsley, parsnip.

Citrus Family: Bergamot, grapefruit, lemon, lime, kumquat, orange, tangerine, and hybrids such as clementine and ugli.

Daisy Family: Artichoke (globe and Jerusalem), burdock, camomile, cardoon, chicory, dandelion, echinacea, endive, feverfew, lettuce, milk thistle, salsify, safflower, sunflower, tarragon.

Goosefoot Family: Beetroot, chard, goosefoot spinach and sugar beet also, but more distantly quinoa.

Grass Family: A large family providing many edible grains. As far as cross reactions go, the following sub-families are more relevant:

1. Barley, kamut, rye, spelt, triticale, wheat (all are gluten grains); but more distantly oats.
2. Corn/maize/sweetcorn, millet, sorghum.
3. Rice, wild rice.

Legume Family: Alfalfa, beans (such as broad, butter, haricot, hyacinth, kidney, lima, mung, runner, soy, but not cocoa), blackgram, carob (locust bean), chickpea, fenugreek, lentil, liquorice, lupin, mangetout, pea, peanut, tamarind and any edible sprouts, such as beansprouts or peanut shoots. Also, legumes used to make additive gums or supplements like acacia, clover, guar, senna, tara, tragacanth.

Lily Family: Aloe vera, asparagus, chives, garlic, leek, onion, shallot, spring onion.

Melon Family: Bitter gourd/karela, cucumber, courgette, gourd (all varieties, including apple, ash and bottle), marrow, melon (all varieties, including honeydew and watermelon), pumpkin, squash, tindori.

Mustard Family: Broccoli, Brussels sprouts, cabbages, cauliflower, Chinese leaf, collard greens, cress, horseradish, kale, kohlrabi (German turnip), mustard, pak choi, radish, rape (canola), rocket, swede (rutabaga), turnip, watercress.

Nightshade Family: Peppers (capsicum and chilli, as well as paprika), physalis (cape gooseberry), potato, tomato; also brinjal/aubergine, but cross reactions with it seem rare.

Rose Family: A large family that gives us many fruits. With regard to cross reactions, these subdivisions are more relevant:

1. Apricot, cherry, damson, greengage, nectarine, peach, plum/prune, sloe, also almond.
2. Apple and pear.
3. Strawberry.
4. Blackberry, raspberry.

Other families

All the above families appear to be the most relevant in food allergic reactions, especially when sensitivity to pollen is involved. The following appear less so, and their members may be less likely to cross react. This is especially true when different parts of the plants are used as food as with the laurels, where fruits (avocado), leaves (bay) and bark (cinnamon) are consumed.

1. Arum family (colocasia, elephant foot yam/aroid, taro/eddo).
2. Cashew family (cashew, mango, pistachio).
3. Currant family (blackcurrant, gooseberry, redcurrant).
·4. Deadnettle family (basil, lavendar, mint, marjoram, oregano, rosemary, sage, thyme, tulsi).
5. Ginger family (cardamom, ginger, turmeric).
6. Knotweed family (buckwheat, rhubarb, sorrel).
7. Laurel family (avocado, bay, camphor, cinnamon).

8. Mulberry family (breadfruit, jackfruit, fig, mulberry).
9. Myrtle family (allspice, clove, eucalyptus, guava).
10. Palm family (coconut, date, palm, saw palmetto).
11. Passion fruit family (passion fruit, granadilla).

Seafood

These divide into three distinct categories namely fish, crustaceans and molluscs, the first and third being sub-divided further.

In general, the closer related any two sea animals are, the more likely you will experience cross reactions between them. In the case of fish, cross reactions between bony fish and cartilagenous fish are the least likely.

Crustaceans and molluscs are often grouped together colloquially as 'shellfish'. There is some evidence that the likelihood of cross reactions between these two groups is higher than that between either group and fish.

Fish

Cartilagenous fish form one class, members are monkfish, ray, shark and skate.

Bony fish form a numerically dominant class, and can be divided into a number of orders, the following of which are the most important:

1. Clupeiformes – anchovy, herring, hilsa, pilchard/sardine, sprat.
2. Gadiformes – cod, haddock, hake, whiting.
3. Perciformes – bass, bream, carangid, croaker, mackerel, perch, red mullet, snapper, swordfish, tilapia, tuna, yellowtail.
4. Pleuronectiformes – flounder, halibut, plaice, sole, turbot.
5. Salmoniformes – pike, salmon, trout, whitefish.

Crustaceans

Crab, crayfish, langouste, lobster, prawn, shrimp.

Molluscs

1. Bivalves – clam, cockle, mussel, oyster, scallop, whelk.
2. Cephalopods – cuttlefish, octopus, squid.
3. Gastropods – abalone, limpet, periwinkle, snail.

Glossary of Allergy Terms

Adrenaline: A hormone which stimulates the cardiovascular system and helps reverse anaphylaxis.

Allergen(ic): (descriptive of) A substance which triggers an allergy in sensitised individuals.

Allergic march: The progression of various allergic diseases as a sufferer goes through childhood, adolescence and then adulthood.

Allergy: A rapid, adverse and inappropriate response of the immune system towards an allergen when it enters the body.

Anaphylaxis: An extreme and dangerous allergic reaction characterised by widespread and alarming symptoms, such as rashes, swellings, difficulty breathing, vomiting, very low blood pressure and loss of consciousness (anaphylactic shock).

Angioedema: Severe swelling and puffiness of the skin, caused by a build up of fluid in deep skin layers.

Antigen(ic): (descriptive of) A substance which is theoretically capable of triggering an allergy in atopic individuals.

Antibody: A protein specifically made by the body to attach itself to and deactivate an allergenic 'invader'.

Antihistamines: Medicines used in the treatment of allergies. They work by blocking the action of histamine.

Asthma: A chronic allergic disease in which the airways (the breathing tubes taking air in and out of the lungs) become inflamed and swollen, making breathing difficult. It is characterised by wheezing and breathing difficulties, and may be aggravated by any number of allergens.

Atopic: (descriptive of) An individual genetically susceptible to allergic illness.

Atopy: An inherited disposition towards allergic illness.

Celiac/coeliac disease: Small intestinal autoimmune disease caused by gluten in the diet.

Cross reaction: Allergic reaction towards an antigenic protein which is similar in chemical structure to one to which the individual is already sensitised.

Dermatitis: Another word for eczema.

Eczema: A chronic allergic disease characterised by severe itching, red rashes, and weeping blisters which become encrusted.

Enzyme: A chemical which brings about a metabolic reaction in the body, typically in relation to digestion or detoxification.

Epinephrine: An alternative name for adrenaline.

Food allergy: Allergy caused by a food constituent, almost invariably a protein within a food, such as a nut or fish protein.

Food aversion: A psychologically based adverse reaction towards a food.

Food (hyper)sensitivity: An umbrella term – either a food intolerance or food allergy.

Food intolerance: A physiological, adverse and delayed reaction to a food or food component which is unlikely to involve the immune system.

Free from food: A food which has been manufactured especially to be 'free from' a particular ingredient or food constituent which may trigger allergies in susceptible people.

Gluten: The dominant protein in wheat, implicated in celiac disease, but also in wheat allergy.

Hay fever: Allergy to plant pollens and spores characterised by sneezing, runny nose and/or nasal congestion, watery eyes, and itching in the nose and eyes, during the pollen season.

Histamine: A chemical released by the body in response to an allergic invader, causing inflammation.

Hives: Another name for urticaria.

Hypoallergenic: (descriptive of) A substance (such as a formula or cream) which is very unlikely to trigger an allergy.

Immune system: The group of cells and organs whose responsibility is to guard against infection and defend the body against attack.

Immunoglobulin: A human antibody.

Immunoglobulin E (IgE): The antibody responsible for classic allergic reactions.

Immunotherapy: A treatment for allergy involving injections or vaccines of tiny amounts of allergen, with a view to desensitising the individual to the allergen.

Oral Allergy Syndrome (OAS): An allergy to fruits, vegetables, herbs, spices and nuts in people with hay fever, caused by cross reactions between pollens and plant foods.

Perennial allergic rhinitis: All year rhinitis, caused by allergy to, for instance, dust mite or pets.

Pollen food syndrome: Another expression for Oral Allergy Syndrome (OAS).

Rhinitis: Inflammation of the lining of the nose, often as a result of airborne allergens.

Seasonal allergic rhinitis: Another term for hay fever.

Urticaria: An allergic reaction characterised by itchiness, wheals and red patchiness of the skin. Also called hives or nettle rash.

Wheal: A bump on the skin characteristic of urticaria, but also indicating an allergic response during a skin prick allergy test (SPT).

Useful Resources

Organisations, medical centres and resources– India

Allergy Asthma Associates: www.allergynasthma.org

Allergy and Asthma Research Centre: www.aarc.co.in

Allergy and Asthma Clinic and Research Center: www.allergyasthmacure.com

Asthma Chest and Allergy Centre: www.acac.in

Bengaluru Allergy Centre: www.bangaloreallergycentre.com

Celiac Society for Delhi: www.celiacsocietyindia.com

Food Safety India: www.foodsafetyindia.nic.in

Food Safety Standards Authority of India: www.fssai.gov.in

Indian College of Allergy, Asthma and Applied Immunology: www.icaai.co.in

The Vegetarian Society: www.vegsocmumbai.com

Food Manufacturers – India

Low-allergen or 'free from' food is likely to increase on the shelves of supermarkets in years to come, especially larger stores, as the import of allergy friendly food from specialist producers in Australia and elsewhere increases. Labelling is likely to be more accurate on products sourced from the West, where strict rules are in place. Some free from food manufacturers based overseas may be willing to ship specialist foods, such as nut-free products, to Asia. The best way to find these is through the web resources or in the magazines listed further below, or you could try asking on an online allergy forum.

There are some specialist producers in India too. Here are a couple.

De'Novo, 315 Industrial Area, Phase 2, Panchkula – 134113, Haryana; telephone: 91-172-259 1125

Gluten-free and wheat-free food products i.e. biscuits, cakes, namkeen, snacks, chocolate, flours, papad, dalia, cake mix, dosa mix and idli mix.

Sunira Foods, 2 Rowland Road, Anand Apartment, Kolkata – 00020; telephone: 33 4008 2638; www.sunirafoods.com

Wheat-free and dairy-free food products i.e. atta, sorghum sooji, dalia, cake mix, brownie mix, pancake mix and cookies.

Medication – India

M K Medical Services: www.mkmedicalservices.com

Asthma and allergy medication

Resources, charities and societies – International

Action Against Allergy (UK): www.actionagainstallergy.co.uk

Allergy and Immunology Society of Thailand: www.immunologythai.org

Allergy Society of South Africa: www.allergysa.org

Allergy UK: www.allergyuk.org

Anaphylaxis Australia: www.allergyfacts.org.au

Anaphylaxis Campaign (UK): www.anaphylaxis.org.uk

American Academy of Allergy Asthma and Immunology:
www.aaaai.org

Asthma UK: www.asthma.org.uk

Australian Society of Clinical Immunology and Allergy (ASCIA):
www.allergy.org.au

British Society for Allergy and Clinical Immunology:
www.bsaci.org

Food Allergy and Anaphylaxis Alliance (US):
www.foodallergyalliance.org

The Food Allergy and Anaphylaxis Network (US):
www.foodallergy.org

Food Allergy Initiative (US): www.faiusa.org

Food Allergy Singapore: www.foodallergysingapore.org

Foods Matter (UK): www.foodsmatter.com

Malaysian Society of Allergy and Immunology:
www.allergymsai.org

National Eczema Association (US): www.nationaleczema.org

World Allergy Organization: www.worldallergy.org

Other useful websites

www.allergicchild.com – support and information resource for families with allergic children.

www.allallergy.net – web portal to a wide selection of online allergy related information, such as articles, journals, publications, resources, data, clinics, products and events.

www.foodallergens.info – food allergy facts, European food allergy information, catering information and more.

www.fooddictionary.eu – food translations in many languages.

www.food-info.net – food composition tables, food allergy advice, and information on reactions to additives and colorings.

www.foodreactions.org – information about all food sensitivities, plus a lively forum.

www.housedustmite.org – information and advice concerning dust mites and allergies.

www.kidswithfoodallergies.org – support and information resource for families with allergic children.

www.latexallergylinks.org – links to latex-allergy related sites across the internet.

Medication – international

ALK Abelló (Denmark). 00 45 4574 7576; www.alk-abello.com

Distributors of the Epipen as well as oral allergy vaccines.

Anapen: www.anapen.com

Epipen. www.epipen.com

Twinject: www.twinject.com

Online discussion/support groups

Internet based forums can offer very good emotional support and information, though some can be unruly at times. Advice is generally well meant, but can never replace authoritative medical opinion. Many are based in the West, so be aware of differences in definitions, healthcare systems and labelling, for instance, when accepting advice. Here are several, but you can find others through some of the resources above, or using a good engine try an internet search ('food allergy discussion' or 'allergy forum', for instance). You could also look on networking sites such as Facebook and search for food allergy groups there.

Allergy Chat: www.allergychat.org/forums

The Food Allergy Kitchen: groups.yahoo.com/group/foodallergykitchen

Food Allergy Survivors Together (FAST): health.groups.yahoo.com/group/fasters

Food Reactions: www.foodreactions.org/forum

Foods Matter Forum: www.foodsmatter.com/foodsmatter_forums/index.php

Peanut Allergy Forum: www.peanutallergy.com/boards

Peanut Allergy UK: www.peanutallergyuk.co.uk

Allergy retailers and manufacturers

There are hundreds of manufacturers and suppliers of allergy products and foods worldwide and many of the resources above have links to a selection of suppliers of items such as translation cards, travel guidebooks, children's products, medical jewellery, medical carrying cases, and much more besides. It is a good idea to 'shop around' a lot before placing an order. To get you started, here are several which are willing to deliver to many international destinations:

Activeaide: www.activeaide.com

Carrying cases, tags and waistbands for injector pens.

Allergy Free Passport: www.allergyfreepassport.com

Translation 'passports' and books for allergy safe travelling and dining; allergy reports and catering advice; food allergy mobile phone applications.

Allergy Grocer: www.allergygrocer.com

Supplies foods guaranteed free from nuts, eggs, soy, wheat, dairy, rice, corn and potato, including beverages, breads, cereals, confectionery, condiments, flours, pastas and snacks.

Kids Alert: www.kidsalert.com.au

Children's T shirts and bracelets carrying allergy warnings.

MedicAlert Foundation: 001 209 668 3333; www.medicalert.org

Charity providing identification bracelets and necklets (Emblems), supported by a 24-hour emergency telephone service in over 100 languages.

Select Wisely: 001 888 396 9260; www.selectwisely.com

Food allergy translation cards in many languages.

Star Allergy Alerts: www.starallergyalerts.com.au

Children's T shirts, stickers, bracelets, badges and other products carrying allergy warnings.

Books

Allergies at Your Fingertips, Joanne Clough (2006, Class Publishing)

How to Manage Your Child's Life-threatening Food Allergies, Linda Marienhoff Coss (2004, Plumtree Press)

The Kid-Friendly Food Allergy Cookbook, Leslie Hammond & Lynne Marie Rominger (2004, Fair Winds Press)

Let's Eat Out with Celiac / Coeliac and Food Allergies!, Kim Koeller and Robert La France (2009, R&R Publishing)

Living with Food Intolerance, Alex Gazzola (2005, Sheldon Press)

The Whole Foods Allergy Cookbook, Cybele Pascal (2005, Whole Foods Publishing)

Magazines

Allergic Living (Canada)
Telephone: 00 1 416 604 0110
Website: *www.allergicliving.com*

Allergy Today (New Zealand)
Telephone: 00 64 9 589 1054

Coping with Allergies and Asthma (US)
Website: *www.copingmag.com/ana*
Telephone: 00 1 615 790 2400

Living Without (US)
Telephone: 00 1 800 474 8614
Website: *www.Livingwithout.com*

Index

A

acupuncture 120

adrenaline 24-39, 155

    care of 31-32

    usage 25-28, 36-38

adrenaline auto-injector pens 26, 162

    care of 31-32

    in pregnancy 38

    risks 37

    usage 26-29, 36-38

alcohol 8, 112, 129

    avoidance 24, 30, 55, 124, 128, 129, 130

    in allergy 13, 76

    intolerance 136

allergic march 3, 155

allergy v-vi *see also* food allergy

    prevalence vi

almond 151 *see also* tree nuts

    foods containing 85

    in cosmetics 68, 69

Anapen *see* adrenaline auto-injector pens

anaphylaxis v, 11-13, 78, 81, 94, 95, 155

    causes 12, 13, 16, 70-71, 137

    children 12, 34-37

    emergency action plans 33-34, 37-38, 76-77

    exercise-induced 12-13, 76

    identification 27, 38

    recovery from 30

    symptoms 11-12, 27, 35-36

    treatment 22, 25-31, 39

angioedema 10, 14, 137, 138, 139, 155

antibodies 2, 156, 157 *see also* IgE antibodies *and/or* IgG antibodies